ALSO BY WALTER M. BORTZ II, M.D.:

We Live Too Short and Die Too Long

DARE to Be 100

Walter M. Bortz II, M.D.

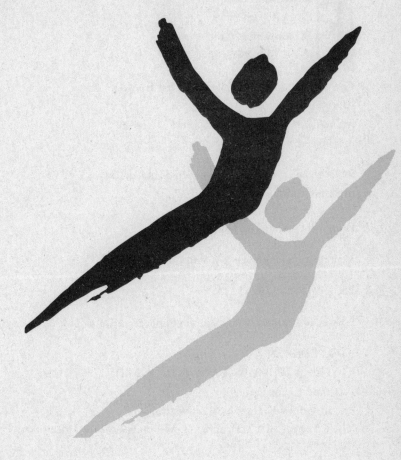

A Fireside Book
Published by Simon & Schuster

FIRESIDE
Rockefeller Center
1230 Avenue of the Americas
New York, NY 10020

FIRESIDE and colophon are registered trademarks
of Simon & Schuster Inc.

Designed by Elina D. Nudelman

Manufactured in the United States of America

20 19 18 17 16 15 14

Library of Congress Cataloging-in-Publication Data

Bortz, Walter M.
     Dare to be 100 / Walter M. Bortz, II, M.D.
          p.   cm.
     Includes bibliographical references.
          1. Longevity.   2. Health.   3. Mental health.   I. Title.
     RA776.75.B67   1996
613'.0438—dc20   96-3260
                                                  CIP

ISBN 0-684-80021-7

This book is dedicated to the thousands of people older than me who have been my teachers. To my parents, to my mentors, but mostly to my patients, almost all of whom are older—many much older—than I. Lessons I learn and have learned from them that I didn't learn in kindergarten: where to seek strength, where to seek peace, and the wisdom to know the difference. Their well-worn lives have provided volumes of instruction and gentle coaching. While the pretense was that I was taking care of my patients, the truth is that they have been taking care of me and nurturing me all along. They have shaped my life, and I am deeply grateful.

Acknowledgments

I wish to express my appreciation first to Jane Gilchrist, with whom the seeds of this book were germinated. I have missed her involvement through its development. I wish further to acknowledge the manuscript preparation assistance of Judy Bentley and the editorial coaching of Judith Durham and Cindy Gitter.

Contents

The Future Isn't What It Used to Be

As we zip along the freeway in our life cruiser, up ahead we see the broadening horizon of January 1, 2000. Entry to a new century is major, no question. But passage to a new millennium is huge. Approaching the wide horizon, we can scarcely help wondering what the terrain up ahead holds. Will the surroundings of January 1, 3000, bear any resemblance to the landscape we are now in? Where will the highway of the next thousand years of human life take us? What are the prominent features of our future maps? Where are the peaks? Where are the valleys? We are traveling so fast now that any speculation is like trying to bring into focus the fleeting images seen through the floor-boards of a moving vehicle. And the speed will only get faster, the picture more obscure and less able to be fixed in our vision.

I was born in 1930, and I recall as a boy hoping that I would live long enough to see the new millennium in—after all, very few have had the chance to live through such an exciting time of giant resetting of calendars and clocks. A lot of zeros will turn over. A new thousand years! It looks like we will have the chance to see what the new Earth time looks like. We are going to live into the next millennium.

As we look ahead, we look, too, out of the corner of our eyes at the rearview mirror and recount where we are coming from. If we strain, we can make out a few traces of the last time a thousand-year calendar turned over. As January 1, 1000, approached, there was fear in the streets. The end of the world was widely forecast. The last judgment was at hand. Superstition, ignorance, and uncertainty were the realities. Europe, in 1000, was in the darkest part of the Dark Ages. Any accounting at that date of the progress since Greek and Roman times would have very few entries.

A thousand years ago, life was tough and crude. Famine and pestilence were everywhere. Average life expectancy was less than twenty years. The Earth was flat. Barbarians roamed freely. The Danes invaded and plundered London. There were eighteen popes in the eleventh century, several succumbing to poison. The estimated world population was 200 million. Leif Erikson visited America around 1000. Chastity belts and suits of armor that would fit only a modern jockey were the costumes. The printing press, the Magna Carta, and the scientific method were still centuries away.

Today's historians have an easy time highlighting achievements from our millennium. But what about the historians of a thousand years from now? How will they rate current Earth time? Without bragging, we can legitimately claim to have come a long, long way in these last ten centuries. In fact, we have come an immense way in the last century alone. Our population approaches 6 billion, thirty times that of a thousand years ago. Life expectancy has risen almost fourfold, jumping thirty years in the last century. Such an increase is represented by the span of time between the Bronze Age and 1900.

We are appropriately told that we live in the Space Age, a term coined the moment we left the gravitational pull of terra firma for the first time to pierce the frontiers of space. Our rearview mirror from that perspective shows the geography of our Earth, which is fully mapped and explored. We have been to the top of the highest mountain and explored the even deeper sea trench off the Marianas Islands. The mirror reveals, too, our history. My mother went to her first job as a schoolteacher in a horse and buggy. I first flew across the country in 1941, in a DC3, stopping at Harrisburg, Pittsburgh, Indianapolis, and then staying overnight in Kansas City before flying on the next day. Now people commute daily from SFO to LAX and from LOG to JFK. The SST allows people to celebrate New Year's Eve on three separate continents. Our rearview mirror provides a look at the recently developed history and geography of the expanding universe, dissection and recombination of the atom, a mapping of DNA, a sequencing of the evolution of life, and a look at the roots of humanity.

All these images and millions more crowd our rearview mirror. They are our landscape and heritage. The history books of A.D. 3000, if they exist, will have a lot to catalog as they survey our era.

Yet there is a contribution of this era that, over future centuries, will have a greater impact on the affairs of this world than all these flashy moments just mentioned. More important than all the space walks, all the computers, and all the Big Macs is the understanding of what a whole human life can look like. The last thousand years have brought unbelievable change. How would the prophets of A.D. 1000 have done predicting today's world? Everything seems so different, but with all the momentous innovations and complexities, one central thing hasn't changed at all—and that is that the DNA, the flesh and putty of which we are made is exactly the same as fifty generations ago. Despite this constancy, and despite all the incredible new knowledge, the notion of just who we are has remained obscure. In his essay "The Future of Man— Evolutionary Aspects," Julian Huxley wrote, "Man's exploration and control of external nature has far outdone his exploration and control of his own nature." The oracle at

Delphi held this precept most sacred: "Know thyself." Despite this exhortation, however, we have had only the vaguest notion of what a whole life could be—until now. It is my firm prediction that it is this new comprehension that holds out the brightest hope for an enriched new millennium. As Huxley goes on to write, "In place of the conflicting areas of the present, our new vision is already indicating the single and over-riding aim of fulfillment. This means greater fulfillment by more individuals and fuller achievement by more societies through greater realization of human possibilities and fuller engagement of human capacities."

Until now, we have not known the extent or content of the human life. Virtually everyone has died too soon, like animals in the wild that rarely have the chance to grow old. The death of a newborn child is so painful because we identify the outrageous cheating of a lifetime. But all premature deaths are outrageous. Peter Laslett wrote, "The greatest part of human life potential has been wasted by people dying before their allotted time was up." The proposition I'm making in this book has never been possible until now, because we haven't had a fix on how long the natural lifespan was.

How long we could or should live has been confused first by the exaggeration of extreme longevity (known as the Methusaleh myth), but even more so by the early deaths of most of the population. The intent of this book is to assert new knowledge about how long we should live, and to explore its immense implications. There is not a feature on this globe or a moment of future time that will be unaffected by this new awareness. It is a noble and hopeful story. It is a happy story. Understanding for the first time in human history what a whole human life can look like is a notion to be cherished and celebrated for as long as our species endures. Old institutions and stereotypes will be challenged and found lacking as a result of this new vision, which allows for the ultimate fulfillment of the human potential.

But the knowledge I impart to you here is not just about the human lifespan. Even richer is the elaboration of the fabric of the life contained between the alpha and omega points. Having the confidence to know where omega is gives great momentum to filling in the rest of the pieces. Put another way, a puzzle is impossible to complete when the horizontal dimension is unknown. When it is secured, the pieces fall naturally into place.

Within this book I intend not only to defend the idea of living to 100, but also to propose the active strategies that will make it happen. As someone wise once noted, "If you are going to get old, you might as well get as old as you can get." The title of this book is an acronym for the steps you need to take to reach 100: D for diet, A for attitude, R for renewal (rest, recreation, retirement, resilience), E for exercise. Three of these components—D, R, and E—are the biological compass points for aiming for 100, but A—attitude—is the most important. Within attitude lie all the planning and decision making that facilitate the biological steps. It is possible to reach 100 by chance, but it's not likely.

It is brilliantly clear that one of life's most precious gifts is the ability to find one's destiny. My mother almost reached 100. She died healthy at 95, with no pills and no infirmity. While her longevity was an accident, yours and mine will be planned. John Lennon said, "Life is what happens to you as you are making other plans." The new science I offer here allows us to be confident and deliberate in our planning. After all, chance favors the prepared person. We not only have that chance, but we also have that responsibility.

This book integrates basic science with philosophy, molecules with wisdom, individual needs with societal concerns, and rights with responsibilities, all in the newly developed time framework of the established expanded human lifespan. It provides a conceptual framework to examine not only what is, but what might be.

Norman Cousins used to tell the story of Johnny, who was a lazy and scatterbrained kid. One day his mother noted that he was quietly and industriously working on something in his room. She called in and asked what he was up to, expecting the worst. Johnny called back that he didn't want to be disturbed, because he was onto something big. Mother couldn't take this evasion, so she barged in to demand an accounting. "If you must know, I'm drawing a picture of God." She retorted, "That sounds like something you would be doing. No one knows what God looks like." Johnny replied, "They will when I get through."

No one has known what life looked like until now. Now we do. Ours is the first generation in history to know what a whole human life can look like. This book shows you that picture.

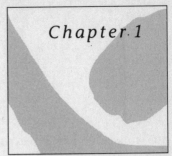

Chapter 1

You've got to have guts to grow old
To claim life you've got to be bold
But you have to be smart
As well as have heart
If you want your whole tale to be told.

Guts and Smarts

In 1995 the first of 75 million baby boomers turned fifty. We know this much. What we don't know is, beginning in 2045, how many of them will turn 100. Two principal credentials will have to be presented if most are to make it—guts and smarts. Smarts is the accumulation and use of the cascade of new knowledge that provides the *when, what,* and *how* to aim for 100. The *when, what,* and *how* involve sorting out and disentangling prior ignorance and misinformation, which has until now prevented full extension of the lifespan. The *when* is the critical appreciation of the dimension of time in everything you do and are. The *what* is the simple assigning of life forces to the proper category, knowing what is changeable and what isn't. And the *how* is the understanding of the way the parts fit together. Our current era is the first in which sufficient knowledge has been accumulated to provide sound answers to these basic questions concerning human life. Having smarts affects each part of your life—the biological, psychological, and social. It affects you individually and collectively as a member of the larger community. It is one of the two basic ingredients of living to be 100.

Smarts	Guts
When	Why
What	
How	

But smarts by themselves aren't enough. Smarts are necessary but insufficient. In order to squeeze all the good out of your life, you also need guts. Guts means having the valor of purpose necessary to pursue the *why*. The capacity to search steadily for a significance in life represents the highest nobility. The *why* is finding a meaning for all of the expanded living and also the energy and involvement necessary to make it happen. Nietzsche is quoted in Viktor Frankl's *Man's Search for Being*: "A person who knows the 'why' of life can put up with almost any 'how.' " For the flame of life to burn brightly for all your days, a steady supply of active participation is essential. If apathy, discontent, and boredom are given room to thrive, your chances of seeing 100 are slim to none. If, however, you muster the guts, nourished by a sense of meaning, then a long vivid life beckons. You need to ensure that each minute of your life is crowded with active participation. It is simply the way nature works, and you need the guts to reach for your natural capacity.

John Gardner suggests that we amend our constitution to read "Life, liberty and the pursuit of meaning." It is the pursuit of meaning that gives life its substance. Without this search we humans are pretty much mindless voyagers on a lonely planet. Yet if we can strive for purpose, then life has a direction. This striving takes guts.

Such heroism does not connote an occasional dash into a burning building or pursuit of other episodic risk of personal safety, but instead reflects a steady, quiet slog across the peaks and valleys of everyday life. Guts and smarts. Courage and intelligence. These are the secrets of the fountain of age, the elixir of a long, bountiful life, the dream of the ancients. Guts and smarts are not mythical, mushy-brained ingredients. They are securely documented, tested, and integrated. They fit precisely into a coherent whole. There is now a sufficient fund of data and experience to allow baby boomers—and, of course, younger generations—to plan their 100th birthday party with calm assurance, prepare the guest list, and muster enough respiratory reserve to blow out all those candles.

But making 100 is not a sure thing. It will not happen effortlessly. It is your job, not someone else's, to see that it happens. As things stand now, the government would hate it, industry would scream, and almost no families would know how to deal with such widespread longevity if we did achieve it. There must be an awful lot of shifting around of old attitudes and social organizations for the boomers and beyond to fit in comfortably as centenarians.

Life inevitably brings losses. The longer you live, the more there will be. The losses themselves are not the principal threat, however. A lack of resilience is. How you confront and adapt to losses is a major ingredient in daring to be 100. There are many pitfalls along the way, disincentives, wrong information, stereotypes, prejudices, and asynchronies. There are many excuses for not wanting to be 100, but they are wrongheaded. The reason all of us should want to live a century are much stronger than the reasons not to. To wish for less than your full potential is dispiriting. We are born for one purpose, and that is to live. When you are ready to die, you must be able to say "Yes, I have lived." Don't spend so much time worrying about whether there is life after death. Worry instead about the life before death.

SMARTS—THE *WHEN*

The first element of developing the smarts necessary for a long life is the new appreciation of the time dimension of your life. How far is it from womb to tomb? An 83-year-old friend of mine told me how he had been more or less looking idly out

the window each day for the undertaker to pull up. Then—
"Eureka!"—he miraculously recognized that "it wasn't time
yet." But until this moment he had lacked the clarity of information to know what stage of life he was living, or put another way, what time it was in his life.

In all likelihood, until now, all of your estimates of your
lifetime have been wrong. How do you know what time it is in
your life? Usually you set your life clock by your parents' and
grandparents' experience. If they died young or old, you more
or less projected that prophecy onto your own life. My maternal grandparents died in their 50s and 60s of cancer and
diabetes, which was pretty much what was expected of them
in the 1920s. My paternal grandparents, however, lived into
their early 70s, and I recall my parents and all of their friends
feeling that Dad's folks were extremely old, outliving their
allotted times. They were in overtime.

I am sure that my parents set their life clocks according to
my paternal grandparents, making midnight for them around
70 years of age. Dad died at 74, just about on cue. But my
mother lived to 95, the last survivor of twelve children, and a
widow for twenty-two years. She was confused and awkward
about her age, despite the fact that she was healthy until she
died. She had lived way past her midnight. On birthdays and
Christmases in our house, she was upset that my kids—her
grandkids—did not turn cartwheels when they found her
check for five dollars in her card. Despite my continued efforts
to encourage her to play a role in our family, she was uncom-
fortable and out of synch. She often told us to "act your age,"
but the problem was that she didn't know how to act *her* age.

Mother lived to 95, not because she paid any heed to the
advice of her physician husband and son. She took perverse
pride in disregarding everything we ever said to her. She was at
least thirty pounds overweight her whole post-me life. Mother
lived to 95 because she was designed to live this long and
longer. We all are.

When my mother was a little girl, the average life expectancy was only 45 years of age. No wonder she felt awfully old near her end. But there is now a virtual consensus that the maximum human lifespan is around 120 years, or one million hours. This does not mean, of course, that all of us will live that long. But at least two people have—Shigecko Isumi was recorded by the *Guiness Book of World Records* as the oldest documented life—120 years, 237 days (but on February 21, 1996, Jean Calment of Arles, France, turned 121). By merely asserting that some of us can live this long creates a noble vision. It is like being President of the United States. Our Constitution asserts that any one of us can be, but very few will. However, the very possibility stretches our imaginations and encourages a sense of participation.

Virtually all biological processes conform to a bell-shaped curve, which is to say that no feature of nature operates in such a way that allows that everyone is the same height or weight, or that all leaves fall off a tree or a shrub on the same day, and so on. In just such a way, natural life expectancy should conform to a bell-shaped curve, the extreme end of which is 120 years. If 120 is the far edge of the curve, where is the center? The answer is 100, meaning that 100 years of age is the median. Ken Manton of Duke University is the leading age demographer in our country. In a recent article in the *International Journal of Forecasting,* he calculated that if the current health habits of the past few years continue, in the year 2080 *the average life expectancy in America will be 100 for men and 103 for women.* Using data supplied by the Census Bureau, Paul Siegel and Cynthia Taeuber predicted that "If the average rates of decrease in death rates continue to prevail in the coming years, in 2050 the average life expectancy will be 100." If this is the case, there will be 19 million centenarians.

These sturdy predictions by leading experts should be heartening for my oldest grandchild, Kellen's, buddies. Three

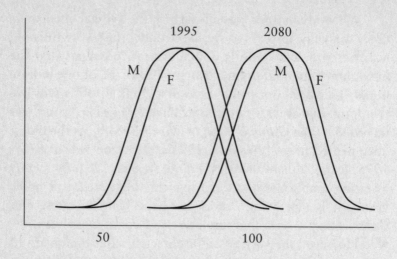

FIG. 1. Average life expectancies between 1995 and 2080.

years ago I gave a very important public address—to his first grade class. Before I started, I passed out papers and asked these bright kids to answer a few basic questions. First I asked how long they would like to live. All but five answered at least 100. One said "forever." The lowest number was 87. Then I asked how long they thought they were going to live. Two answered less than 80, six answered 80 to 90, four answered 90 to 100, the other ten answered 100 plus, one 125, another 254.

A year or so ago, the Alliance for Aging Research conducted a man-on-the-street survey and asked essentially the same questions. Two thirds of the people, this time adults, also said they wished they could be 100 if—and this is the important if—they could stay healthy.

Given this data, we now know how to set our watches and clocks and calendars. Midnight on the 31st of December comes at 120 years of age. For a 30-year-old that means he or she is only at three o'clock, or in March of the year. A 60-year-old is at six o'clock, or in June. Not until older ages does winter set in. Knowing how to "time" lifetimes is surely one of the most powerful tools we can use to live a fulfilled life. It is a key component of smarts. The *when* of life.

The physicists teach us that there are really only three basic components of the universe: matter, energy, and time. We mortals can have some input into the first two of these, matter and energy, but time is beyond our control. No one has yet found out how to alter time. This is clear. What isn't clear is our ability to know which aspects of our lives are controlled by the effects of time, over which we have no influence, and which are due to the interaction of energy and matter, which we can actively confront. The distinction between these two aspects is one of the great benefits of being able to comprehend the true time boundaries of our lives.

Until now, we have understood only two times of life, youth and adulthood. Youth and adulthood were and are extremely well studied and understood. There are innumerable texts describing in abundant detail what being a child and an adult are all about. Being a child means growth, learning, developing, maturing. Adulthood means childbearing and -rearing, the time of work. What comes next? The answer for most people, until relatively recently, is that they die. But when you realize that there are as many people alive over 65 years of age in the world today as in all previous history put together, you get the idea that the opportunity to grow old—to live into a new third age of life—has only rarely existed before. Now it is common and becoming more so, as 15 percent of women and 4 percent of men now live into their nineties. The most rapidly growing segment of the American population is the centenarians, not because of any great medical breakthroughs, but simply because they, like my mother, are fulfilling their natural biological heritage.

Having the smarts to understand the true time dimension of life can be powerfully shaping. With this knowledge, you can redesign your life. Such a positive act helps offset what psychologist Martin Seligman calls "the helpless-hopeless" syndrome.

Numerous examples exist that indicate that for many people death seems to occur on cue. Voodoo death and the pointing of the bone are vivid evidences of negative predictions. There are, as well, positive examples in which people die at lower than predicted rates in periods immediately before important holidays or celebratory events. For example, elderly Chinese die at lower than expected rates in the period preceding the Moon Festival and higher rates immediately thereafter.

With a foreshortened lifespan expectation, how can you logically plan the last of your new life? How can you see and know the whole when only the first part has been studied? How can you understand a novel, a mystery, a movie, a ballgame if you leave part of the way through? Now that we see the last part, we can understand the whole.

As children we presume that most of our life will be spent going to school. As young adults we presume that most of our life will be spent with children in the house. As working people we presume that most of our life will be spent working. All wrong. Life is made up of these segments, but the huge postworking segment is unaccounted for. Is it possible that this last segment is the longest of all? What is the job description of this new-found lifetime? It is a gift of found time.

Lack of sensitivity to this time dimension of life leads naturally to an assertion of immediate self-gratification—the newborn baby has no patience. If there is no sense of tomorrow, we naturally want it all today. If life is going to last 40, 60, or 80 years, we need to get it all done in that span.

What if it were possible to know exactly how long we were going to live? What if our birth certificate had an expiration date stamped on it? The lifestyle of the inner city toughs is predicated on having no life calendar. Each day has no future. Logic is irrelevant—all because of lack of identification and appreciation of a sense of lifetime. If gang members knew with confidence that they could and would live to be 100, their mad pursuit of consumption and immediate gratification and glory would erode. Length of life has consistently been shown to relate to intelligence in general. And length of life should logically be expected to relate very highly to intelligence about how long a person might live!

The point is, we can play an active role in determining our lifespan, as long as we understand that it is mutable and not fixed. Having established reliably our true lifetime potential is one of the most precious intellectual gifts our species will ever receive. But of equal or even greater importance is the nature of the new longer life, the *what* and the *how*.

SMARTS—THE *WHAT*

Marie Garibaldi is the chief justice of the New Jersey Supreme Court. In 1987 she wrote an opinion in the matter of Kathleen Farrell. The case involved the issue of whether life support efforts could or should be withdrawn from Farrell, a 37-year-old competent, terminally ill patient suffering from ALS, commonly known as Lou Gehrig's disease. Her life was being artifically sustained in the intensive care unit by means of major medical technology. Justice Garibaldi wrote, *"Matters of fate have become matters of choice."* In this simple sentence she captured the essence of the illuminating moment in mankind's history. Until recently, death was random and virtually immutable. Fate ruled, and what happened was not ours to anticipate or challenge. Even twenty years ago, Kathleen Farrell would not, could not, have lived. Of course, recent knowledge and technology have changed that.

The shift of human destiny from fate to choice is enabled by one thing, and that is knowledge. For the first time we have enough smarts to propose a coherent whole view of what life can look like. We know how long it can be (the *when*) and, significantly, the nature and course of those conditions that threaten its quality as well as extent. We don't enter the future; we create it.

Along the same lines, almost everything in the medical textbooks about aging is wrong, inadvertently confusing one disease or condition with one another, and often returning to the presumption that aging by itself is the villain. The hackneyed joke concerns the old fellow with the sore leg visiting the doctor's office. The doctor, after a cursory exam, attributes the sore leg to aging. The patient's challenge—"But, Doc, the other leg is just as old and it's fine"—is haunting. Sure, aging and the passage of time play a role, but not nearly to the extent that have been presumed until now. This is great news. For conditions of old people not to be due to the passage of time gives hope that counterstrategies can be derived to prevent or reverse at least a major part of them. As we develop a conceptual framework of what aging truly is, we become newly able to reformulate the whole of the conditions that affect our lives.

FATE VS. CHOICE

Fate ⟶ Choice

Conditions as diverse as tuberculosis, hardening of the arteries, and Alzheimer's disease have in the past fatefully been conceded by practitioners to be due to aging. The error in this miscategorization is now clear, but as recently as forty-five years ago, stiff and clogged arteries were thought by all to be a reflection of "God's will." It is now evident that this fatalism was wrong. The facts that young people have some arteriosclerosis, that some old people don't, and that it is reversible proves that the condition is not due to aging. What this tells us is that it is susceptible to control.

By putting the correct label of disease on arteriosclerosis, fate is replaced by the choices of prevention or treatment. Medicine, like politics, is based on the art of the possible. If an illness is acknowledged to be due to something that is either obscure or beyond one's control, then little effort is likely to be expended.

But what if the illness is not inscrutable, and a curing moment is lost because of the application of the wrong tag?

The correct diagnosis has been the cornerstone of the practice of medicine. When the cause of a condition is accurately known, the precision of treatment is made possible. Medicine has labored long and hard to make diagnosis and the rational categorization of disease a science. In my grandparents' day, thousands of people died of "acute indigestion." Thousands die today of "myocardial infarction," the same condition, but under the correct explanation.

Much confusion streams from the lack of a lifetime perspective. Illnesses are still viewed as static episodic events. This snapshot approach is driven, too, by the "quick fix" urgency of high medical costs. The acute moment of the illness obscures the evidence of earlier excess spending. In other words, only when the check bounces does an overdraw and sick notice arrive. Additionally, too much faith in the power of technology to cure has seduced us into unsound health practices.

Aging, too, has lacked a conceptual framework. By and large it has been neglected as a legitimate target for scientific study, or worse, it has been slotted as a traditional disease like scarlet fever, thereby susceptible to a curative approach. Where does aging come in? Does it deserve a subheading under all other headings, is it a disease, a process, a behavior, a symptom? What exactly is aging? Most texts don't even try to define it. Many describe symptoms that are commonly found in old persons, but almost none make an effort to provide a conceptual framework into which aging fits.

This is one of the intellectual gifts given to medicine by new research with old people. Conditions can be placed in the right slots.

This new formulation proposes that all human ailments fall into four separate and distinct types. Not only do these types have different causations, but their causations also lead to specific approaches, and even further to specific and appropriate public policy responses. These four types are (I) blue-print error, (II) lightning, (III) dissonance, and (IV) time. In more technical language, they are conditions of genetic defect, extrinsic agency, intrinsic agency, and aging.

BLUEPRINT ERROR

If I, and you, have heard it once, we have heard it a thousand times. "If you want to live to a ripe old age, be sure to choose old grandparents." Cute, but wrong. Heredity has little to do with how long you live. Many scientific studies, including those which study longevity records of twins, conclude that inheritance has only 15 to 20 percent to do with how long you will live. In other words, "It's not the cards you're dealt that matter most, it's how you play your hand."

Certainly there are conditions due to a bad blueprint. These are known as the genetic diseases, such as sickle-cell anemia and cystic fibrosis, which clearly are the result of mismatched or defective genes and chromosomes. For-tunately, most bad seeds are expelled in utero, yet some do survive. Most mismatches that make it to the world are prob-lems of early life, encountered largely by pediatricians. Once you make it to midlife, the medical conditions are basically not those due to defective design, but to conditions over which you can exercise a high degree of personal control.

The reason this is so important to emphasize is that until now people have, fatalistically, more or less programmed their health as an issue presided over largely by one's grandparents, and if a problem arose, the doctor would rush right in to restore order. It's not that simple.

LIGHTNING

Until the present era, nearly all deaths were caused by light-ning conditions—meaning conditions in which the person afflicted had little or no role to play in their occurrence. Such conditions are infections, malignancies, injuries, poisonings, and war. At the start of this century, eight of the top killers were lightning conditions—pneumonia, meningitis, tuberculosis, and so on. Virtually the entire current medical establishment has been dedicated to addressing lightning conditions, antibiotics and surgery being the two principal areas developed to offset them, exemplified by removal of a tumor or the administration of penicillin for a strep throat. Most medical technology and efforts of the pharmaceutical industry are directed to curative approaches to these events.

Importantly, lightning conditions often lend themselves to a curative effort. Time usually has played no role in the event, and the afflicted person can, by a direct and specifically targeted therapy, be restored to the original state of health. Much great good has occurred as a result of our new understanding and treatment of lightning conditions. Unfortunately, however, new villains have rushed upon the stage, and it is these conditions, which are due to dissonance, that now crowd doctors' offices and hospitals.

DISSONANCE

Unlike lightning conditions, in which the individual has little or no personal role to play in the ailment, dissonance conditions are the direct result of the inappropriate relationship of the person with his or her environment. Further, their onset is insidious, they take years to develop, and once encountered do not lend themselves easily to cure. This is not to say that heroic amounts of energy and money aren't spent in the effort, but like Humpty Dumpty, once the cracks are made, cure is impossible. Heart attacks, strokes, arthritis, emphysema, and cirrhosis are common examples of medical conditions due to dissonance, or imbalance.

Dissonance comes in two varieties: too much and too

little. Too much contact between the environment and the individual is known as stress; too little as disuse. Stress is an epidemic condition in which a person suffers a broad array of physical problems as the result of what Stanford physicist William Tiller calls the "high event density of life"—constant bombardment by a tremendous assortment of often unpleasant and noxious stimuli. Ulcers, high blood pressure, diabetes, kidney damage, and skeletal and emotional problems result from living in a world that often seems simply to be spinning too fast. Disuse, on the other hand, leads to a long list of problems, including cardiovascular vulnerability and musculoskeletal fragility, as the direct byproduct of insufficient stimulation of our bodies by physical inactivity. What I, and other doctors, see in our offices is usually a result of a mixture of these two kinds of dissonance. Our brains are frizzed by too much energy, while our bodies shrivel because of too little stimulation and exercise.

Sixty years ago, famed Harvard professor Walter Cannon coined the useful term "homeostasis" to indicate the wonderful ability the body exhibits to maintain its equilibrium when buffeted by too many or too few influences. Our homeostatic mechanisms allow us to function in the heat and cold, dark and light, fed and starved, at rest and under heavy workloads. Dissonance conditions occur when these stabilizing devices are tested beyond their ability to compensate.

TIME

Finally, we come to aging. We have until recently lacked a good definition of aging, and as a result we have assigned too much mischief to it. It is not an exaggeration to assert that almost everything we have been taught about aging has been wrong. Casually and wrongly, we have catalogued almost everything that happened to an older person as due to the passage of time. The truth is that until recently we haven't lived long enough to die of aging. Virtually everything that has been consigned to aging is due instead to the accumulation of changes due to lightning and dissonance.

This recognition is absolutely critical. Aging, in my definition, is the effect of an energy flow on matter over time. It is inevitable and nonpreventable. The march of time leads to the gradual accumulation in all our selves of debris, trash, the result of the generation by our metabolism of free radicals. But as we will learn in the next chapter, aging proceeds at a more stately pace than has originally been thought.

Four possible survival curves of a hundred coffee mugs in the dishwasher are represented in figure 2 on page 32. They conform to the four categories just described. In scenario A nearly all cups break the first day, because they just weren't made to last in the hubbub of the dishwasher. In scenario B all cups break randomly, one each day by accident. The graph looks like the human survival curve of 1900. In scenario C the cups don't break until after fifty days, when assorted minor nicks and cracks accumulated over the first weeks add up and breakage appears. This curve represents the survival curve symbolic of human lifespans. Finally, in scenario D, all cups break on the last day because they simply wore out. This is what engineers call systems death. The first three scenarios represent death from component failure, one or another isolated breakdown leading to death, while the rest of the organism is still okay. Very few of us have lived long enough to get to scenario D. But we will.

This new formulation of the four types of agencies that affect not just the length of our lives but also their quality is made possible by the identification of the power of time in human affairs. If life is viewed as nothing more than a series of unconnected snapshots, then this reconceptualization is impossible. But when we understand life as a long set of tightly connected and interdependent processes, this new comprehension is made possible.

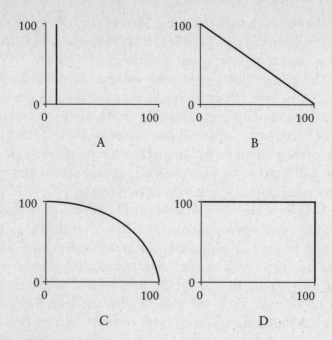

FIG. 2. Coffee cups and us. Four survival scenarios.

From this definition it is possible to create effective therapies. Blueprint error and time are fate, agencies beyond easy approach. But both lightning and dissonance are phenomena that lend themselves powerfully to preventive and corrective strategies: choice. This differentiation is made possible by the proper redefinition of aging.

OTHER REDEFINITIONS

Not only does the comprehension of the true time of a lifetime, the *when*, lead to a deconstruction and reconstruction of the health and medical care system, but it leads inevitably to scrutiny of other basic institutions of our society.

Many of our oldest institutions are out of date. They were formulated centuries ago when our ancestors died in their 40s,

50s, and 60s, yet we have made little effort to correct them. Now it is clear that we must, if we are to survive with any sense in the system, presuming we have the smarts to do it.

The educational system, the work career, and the basic family organization are fundamental social constructions that must be reexamined in the light of our new knowledge about the human lifespan. There is invariably a substantial lag phase between the occurrence of any major novel event—such as a new technology or catastrophe or demographic shift—and the impact on the persons involved. The arrival of tens of millions of baby boomers into newly extended lifetimes predictably will cause substantial political, economic, and personal unrest—until the new realities are recognized, analyzed, and reacted to.

The arrival of the baby boomers at the third stage of their lives represents a disruptive occasion. This huge age cohort has already been held accountable for many changes in the educational system in America. It has been claimed that when this group attained school age, in 1951, the schools changed from being educational institutions to child care centers, simply because there weren't enough teachers and school monies available to accommodate the glut of new students. Similarly, their arrival into the housing market resulted in the boom in real estate prices in the 70s.

This gang exits their work phase to what? What are the opportunity structures out there to meet them? There appears to be a large gap between the potential of 100-plus years and the tasks that the new design offers. Lacking opportunity, the tens of millions of newly old will find a roleless role to play, a process that has been termed "social death."

Sociologists John and Mathilda Reilly explain that the rigid age-defined sequence of education, work, and leisure was developed when life expectancy was only 45 years of age, and it was developed largely as a male model. But what seems needed now is an age-integrated approach, in which educa-

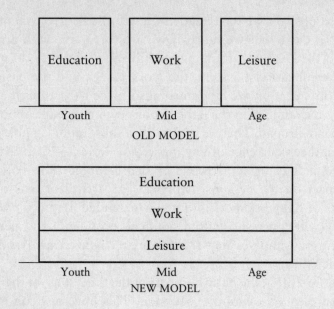

FIG. 3. Life Phases.

tion, work, and leisure are distributed over the lifespan—a model that more closely approximates a female life strategy. Each life phase should include elements of each function.

Of course, we need the smarts to carry this off, including field experiments, to see how each function fits into each life phase.

LIFELONG LEARNING

Knowledge is said to double every seven to ten years. What if you stop learning around 20 years of age, and live another eighty years thereafter, with no further educational pursuit? This scenario clearly makes no sense. Our present system of grade school, junior high, high school, college, and the rest was instituted back in Elizabethan times when life expectancy was about 35. It probably made sense then to matriculate until the early twenties and then go to work, hope for a decade or so of work, and then die. But what about now, as we reach to 100? Is it right to read your last book at age 22 and then live eight more decades without any formal effort to rev up your brain?

Gerhard Casper, president of Stanford University, is known for his enthusiasm for shortening the college curriculum from four years to three as a cost-cutting measure. I propose an alternative scheme: instead of shortening the study course to three years, expand it to eighty. As a freshman is admitted at age 18, he or she is enrolled in a program that has study courses every so often and culminates in graduation around age 98. Others have suggested taking every tenth year off from work for an educational boost. The sabbatical model makes a lot of sense from many perspectives.

What does a lifelong learning curriculum look like? Clearly, no single formula is appropriate for all. Emphasis on maintaining and extending cultural tradition, enrichment of historical perspectives, and libraries would perpetuate the social role that elders have played in society since the earliest times. Many formats will be necessary to encompass the needs of those persons with mobility or other frailty concerns. No one is ever too old to learn. The Elderhostel movement is booming. Its 1994 catalog listed more than 10,000 programs.

The necessity of reorganizing our educational institutions in the face of a lifetime of 100 years cuts directly to the heart of the issue as to whether the last fifty years of life is spent as a liability or as a resource. As the huge cohort of baby boomers turning 50 confronts what is left for them in life, how educated they continue to be is a critical and society-shaping issue. If they remain content to coast on knowledge gained in their first two decades, their role as social burdens will be assured. However, if somehow there can be a consensus built that education is a continuing responsibility, then the scene is set for the omega generations to claim their appropriate role as vital, contributing, abundant segments of the larger community. While an educated elder is a precious resource, a disconnected, disinterested, disused elder is a liability. The newly identified life expectancy demands a redesigned educational format so that lifelong learning is facilitated and rewarded.

WORK MATTERS

As a longer lifespan mandates reexamination of early life and its commitment to learning, so, too, does it force a rethinking of work time. Retirement in the mid-60s was appropriate when first initiated a hundred years ago in Germany. Very few people even lived long enough to reach retirement then. But now, many people spend almost as much of their lives post-retirement as when working. This 65th birthday is sanctified as a major life marker, an event which my Palo Alto Clinic mentor, Dr. Russel Lee, liked to call "statutory senility." The event usually signals a major downshifting of gears from participating to spectating, simply because of a calendar date that has absolutely no biological significance.

In 1900 67 percent of men over 65 worked; in 1950 half did. Now, fewer than one sixth do. From an era derived during Puritan time, in which work was judged to be essential for self-esteem ("don't outlive your work"), we enter a time in which workers see retirement as a right earned after a life of work at the bench. A state of structured dependency is the result.

The new availability of generous social security and employer pension benefits are seductions to an early retirement. Social security payments rose from $5 billion in 1950 to $250 billion in 1990, from 2 to 20 percent of federal spending. This clearly can't go on.

The new abundant leisure time afforded by retirement is dangerous. One fourth of retirees admit to a feeling of obsolescence, completely separate from the notion of money. The

Gallup organization asked a number of older volunteers how they got started. "Someone asked," was the common reply. The opportunity for important volunteer work gratifies the need to be valuable. Thirty-six percent of people over 55 do volunteer work, but 40 percent more say they would like to. They need only be enlisted.

New work formats need to evolve. The forty-hour work week with two weeks off in the summer as vacation just won't cut it. More flexible schedules relating to retraining and reeducation, job shifts, expansion of career options, and creation of interchangeable responsibilities are consistent with the redefinition of our work experience. For many, life is defined by work. If this is true, a radical redefinition is in order, in light of our longer and healthier lifespans.

FAMILY MATTERS

The opportunity to confidently predict and live a hundred years places the family in a different context. The future necessitates that all of us be prepared for remaining vitally involved with the family structure. Of course, this means that there must be roles to play and responsibilities to fulfill. One hundred years of life means at least four generations, and maybe even five. The sandwich generations—and the first generations as well—should profit from the presence and wisdom of the older generations. The elders of the family are, for better or worse, prophets to the younger generations about what their future may hold. Our frenetic domestic mobility has devalued the role of the family elders, but many studies indicate that being near family is one of the most highly desired elements of retired persons. In fact, various research reports validate that people who retain family relationships live longer and are more functional. In other words, social ties double survival.

It is certainly true that the stereotypical family unit has

many new and complex variations. New devotions and affilia-
tions arise, and many families are geographically scattered.
The resulting erosion of interdependence among kin leads to
insecurity and isolation in old age. Notable, too, is the trend
toward government, as opposed to family, responsibility for
the well-being of older people as usually this surrogate governmental support is both economically insufficient and lacking
in emotional sustenance.

Regular communication, the sharing of goods and ideas,
maintenance of tradition, and mutuality of support efforts are
all components of family life that aid in longevity. The proposition that all of us can and should live to 100 opens up the
possibility for family role playing. It endorses the idea that the
best way to make the new design fulfilling is within the family
framework—all for one, one for all.

Guts and smarts are the ground rules for 100. This chapter has as its central intent the establishment of the horizontal
time dimension of the life portrait, the *when,* and assignment
of its ingredients to the proper category—fate versus choice,
the *what.* Loudly proclaimed these days are "right to die"
initiatives. But rights derive from responsibility. Yes, we all
have the right to die, but only after having lived responsibly.
We now know enough that this responsibility is here to stay.
The ability to distinguish what is ours to choose and change,
and what is ours to accept, has been sacred since St. Francis
and before. The *when* and *what* of smarts lead naturally to the
how, which is the subject of the next chapter.

Chapter 2

Our "Just So Story," or How We Got This Way

Hamlet was partially right. *"To be or not to be"* is still a substantial question, but *how* to be is at least as important. The *how* of life determines the *whether*. The easy explanation for the *how* of life is that an egg and a sperm happily match up, mix up their nucleotides, and make their baby, or chick, or seedling. After the union the offspring, whatever it is, grows up and goes merrily on its way until it runs out of steam and dies, carefree and mindless and effortless. Fate takes over.

But just a minute, it's not that simple. For almost all of the animal world, nothing dies a natural death. The *how* of life is determined almost exclusively by getting enough to eat (and not being eaten) and avoiding being struck by lightning. In this regard, we humans are continually unique. The daffodil or zebra has little choice about how it, he, or she interacts with its environment. There is no choice; there are no options. Survival depends on luck, whether good or bad. We, on the other hand, have virtually limitless options as to how to live our lives, and yet we seem to exhibit a remarkable ability to self-destruct. Such behavior is inexcusable. When you deal with dying patients, as I do every day, you see many of their desperate efforts to stay alive, to buy another ounce of time. Meanwhile, you witness another person flaunting his or her lifetime endowment and engaging in reckless self-abuse. I acknowledge that most self-abusers don't know any better, but their excuses are no longer acceptable. Until recently our information base was insufficient to make defensible choices about *how* to live, but now all the parts of these strategies are there for every one of us to see, learn, and respect.

Your body has a certain energy content. If you presume a daily food intake that contains 2,000 calories, that calculates out to one sixty-fifth of a body's worth of energy. Said in another way, the body totally replaces—or remakes—itself at the caloric level every sixty-five days (or roughly six times a year). On a whole-life basis, a daily caloric food intake of 2,000 calories × 100 years = 73 million calories that go in your mouth over a lifetime. That is to say, you consume 600 bodies' worth of energy over a lifetime.

These calculations are intended to emphasize that your body is constantly changing, even though the mirror doesn't show it. You are not the same person as last year or next year. Tomorrow is different. Of course, not all of the body replaces itself at the same rate. The body is in constant flux and every one of your 1,000 million million cells and 1,000 million million million million atoms is changing minute by minute, all under the control of mechanisms that are just starting to be understood.

THE *HOW* OF DEVELOPMENT

The last twenty years have seen an immense surge in the scientific understanding of the mechanisms behind development. One of my favorite organisms is the Lonesome Cypress on the gorgeous 17-Mile Drive in Carmel, California. Celebrated on millions of calendars and postcards, its shape has been recast to reflect the westerly winds that changed it from a straight-up cypress to one that lists sharply to the east. Its DNA said "straight," but the wind said "east."

An extended example of the interplay of form and environment is a forty-year experiment still in progress here at Stanford by a series of scientists. These workers, supported by the Carnegie Foundation, planted plants of the same mustard weed species in different locations, from the Pacific shoreline to the crests of the Sierra Mountains. The plants, just like those in your backyard or park, assume a wide variety of shapes and forms, depending on where they are planted. They become where they live.

Each of the 650,000 species of plants must be adaptable to the environment, even more than their animal cousins. The reason for this, of course, is that animals possess the advantage of movement, meaning that they can change location to conform to their environmental preferences, unlike their plant relatives, which are moored to one spot. Plants must respond to changes in temperature, moisture, sunlight, and mechanical pressure. Cellulose, "the beams of plants," has the highest strength to density ratio known in nature. Applying a weight to a plant stem for forty-eight hours leads to a strength that is twice the breaking force. As a fruit stretches its stem, the strength increases a thousandfold. Plants exposed to wind have shorter and thicker stems. Experimenters have unexpectedly discovered that the measuring of plants stunts their vertical growth. Merely touching or blowing on or spraying the plant Arabidopsis creates changes in the genes of the plants within minutes. The levels of messenger RNA that control cell growth go up a hundredfold within ten minutes of stimulation and stay up for one to two hours. Touching the plant sets in motion a sequence that changes the structure-making apparatus of the plant to conform to the stimulus. This is the molecular translation of how the environment shapes form. This is the "just so story" of how the Lonesome Cypress got its shape.

Every cell in the animal world is likewise impacted by its environment and reacts and conforms to the specific demands, and it is the musculoskeletal system that is the most thoroughly studied. Studies of prehistoric bones reveal ridges and grooves that indicate that the lifestyle of these creatures was much more vigorous than ours. Our weak bones, the result of our inactive lives, lead to the epidemic condition of osteoporosis and the hundreds of thousands of hip, pelvis, and spinal fractures suffered each year. It is interesting to observe that right-handed tennis players have much larger muscles and denser bones in the right arm than in the left.

But maybe more important to our survival is the effect of use on our arteries. Heart disease is more properly known as artery disease. It is far and away our biggest killer. What is the effect of use on arteries? Our research group looked at the size of the heart and coronary arteries in a group of endurance athletes and found that these tubes were substantially bigger than those of inactive persons. Similarly, bicyclists have been shown to have larger arteries to their legs, whereas those to their arms and head are no different from those of inactive people. This structural change has now been decoded to show how an increased flow through an artery actually leads to changes in the genetic machinery leading to bigger arteries. The lesson: We actually become what we do.

THE MECHANISM OF DEVELOPMENT

This new information allows a presentation of how nature acts to conform structure to function. Every cell in nature has on its surface thousands of antennae, which the biochemists call receptor sites. These antennae function to catch energy. Like the TV aerial, they catch what is nearby. There are several types of receptors. Some catch radiant energy as light (the retina); some catch sound energy (ear); some catch heat, cold, acid, sweet, electric, pressure, and so on. Even intestinal cells have mechanoreceptors, which sense the pushes and pulls in the gut and conform their structure to the pressure, just like the plant stem.

In essence, the message is that the hardware of life is less important to our lifelong well-being than is the software. The program is the message. And this is good news, because it means that we are not confined to a life pattern preordained by forces over which we have no control. Our birth was someone else's doing, and our death is an eventual byproduct of being alive; these facts are fated. But the content and extent of the life from alpha to omega is largely ours to shape.

The fact that our environment makes so much difference to our body's effectiveness makes a lot of sense. Linking the structure of any one of us or any part of us to the environment creates a functional bonding that a blueprint alone can't provide, allowing for speedy and appropriate repair if injury should occur.

Study of the processes of development clearly shows that growth is not confined to the first part of life. It is a lifelong affair. When a shrub or tree stops growing, it dies. It needs to reach toward and touch the sunlight from which it derives its energy and structure. No energy, no form. Another way to put it is "Use it or lose it."

While the rest of nature lacks the information to make optimal its relationship with its habitat (and therefore, the fit is decreed by circumstance), for humans, survival no longer depends on luck and instinct. It depends, instead, on our skill at profiting from these lessons. Our bodies have optimal operational ranges. We need to see that they are run within this range—not above or below—if our 100-plus years are to be sustainably vital. Fate is replaced by choice, as we grasp how the universe in general—and ourselves in particular—work.

FRAILTY

Understanding of the basis for developmental process gives entry to the consideration of frailty. Like aging, frailty has lacked a conceptual framework. Is frailty a disease? If it is, where do we look for it in our medical classrooms or text-books? Is frailty a legitimate entry on a death certificate? Can I admit one of my patients to Stanford Hospital with just the diagnosis of frailty, and if I can will the insurance company pay for it?

Or is frailty aging? Its appearance mostly in old persons seems to indicate that time has something to do with the frailty. But we can quickly identify young people who are frail as a result of multiple causes, malnutrition prime among them. Therefore, frailty is not synonymous with aging. Even more important is the central observation that even 90-year-olds can recapture lost vigor with an exercise program. Just what, then, is frailty? It is the reciprocal of vitality, robustness, and healthiness. It is a predisposition to failure. It is a disconnec-tedness, a weakness, an infirmity.

FRAILTY AND MEDICAL CONDITIONS

In more scientific terms, frailty is a downward drift of matter from a more highly organized state of order, structure, and function to a state of increased disorder, instability, and sus-ceptibility. The cause of this total decay is the loss of contact of the system from its environment, with its ordering capacity. The sources of this loss of contact between the organism and its environment lie in each of the four categories of illness described earlier: blueprint error, lightning, dissonance, and time. Blueprint error results in malfunctioning infants with predispositions to problems. Lightning leads to frailty as a result of scars and accumulated debilities. Aging, too, contrib-utes to frailty, as the wear and tear of metabolism exerts its toll. Of course, a 90-year-old is not the same person as a 20-year-old. But it is in the area of dissonance—conditions of intrinsic agency—where frailty finds its principal expression. In 1900 people died at the average age of 45 of type II conditions (lightning), whereas now the average age is 75, and type III conditions (dissonance) are largely the reason. If we aspire to reach 100, to have the chance to die of aging, we must address the dissonance conditions—those caused by faulty relationships with the environment—and the resulting frailty and chronic disease states that are killing us now. The progressive development of frailty also leads to increased susceptibility to lightning conditions. At 30 we can withstand a fractured hip easily; at 90 a fractured hip can be fatal.

My personal attention to frailty was derived from the result of a ski accident thirty years ago. I ruptured the Achilles tendon on my right ankle. I rode the ski patrol toboggan to the bottom of the slope, enduring the good-natured kidding by my children about their awkward father. Eventually, the tendon was resutured and my leg put in a plaster cast for six weeks. When it emerged, it was withered, purple, and painful—not because it was old, or even because it was operated on, but because it had been in a cast. Frailty results from disuse—even more than it does from aging.

Frailty represents a diminished level of function. It is not a disease. It is a condition—a too-common condition that has previously lacked definition. It is not in the medical textbooks. It is not in the handbook of diagnoses of the World Health Organization. The Health Financing apparatus does not recognize it as a legitimate reason for hospitalization. Yet it appears as a huge and overlooked reality.

It is also critical to observe that frailty is not aging. Some young people, like my leg in a cast, develop frailty. Further, it is reversible, no matter at what age. But how can we sort out what is frailty due to blueprint error, lightning, or dissonance?

How much of the decrepitude of older people is due to time's ravages, and how much is due to other preventable causes?

To sort these issues out, my son Walter (a doctor) and I reviewed a number of records from athletic events—running, rowing, and swimming. We found that over time, performances in these events declined at ½ percent per year. We concluded, therefore, that no single vital function can deteriorate from age—or anything else—faster than this rate if the performance is to be sustained.

I believe, therefore, that ½ percent per year is a vitally important number. This is *the* central biomarker of true age changes. The ½ percent per year value happens to correspond with a wide range of body functions not associated with exercise performance such as cognitive change, wound repair, telomerase levels (a basic gene control enzyme), nail growth, or skeletal calcium loss. We proclaim that true age change equals ½ percent per year. Anything faster than this is not aging—and therefore is susceptible to intervention.

Now back to the vitality-fragility scale. If we presume that at age 30 we have maximum vitality and then, like Archie Bunker, we start to surrender 2 percent per year, by age 65 we become frail (35 years × 2 percent per year = 70 percent lost, which by definition is frailty). This calculation closely mimics the observed high incidence of frailty in those above 65 years of age, even in the absence of categorical disease. If, on the other hand, you maintain your best function and decay at the rate of ½ percent per year, at age 65 you have surrendered only 15 percent of original vitality, and virtually full functional capacity is assured. Extrapolation of these figures indicates that frailty might never be encountered before age 120, the biological age limit. We want to die healthy. Such extrapolation is only theoretical because these observations hold only until the 70s, at which point records start to deteriorate. It may be that the ½ percent per year is a linear function through the middle years but could become greater later on, so that

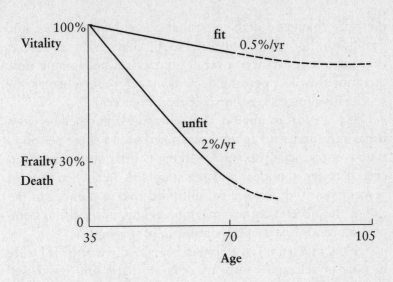

FIG. 4. Age and Vitality.

frailty may accelerate in the 90s or later, but this theory is speculative.

A critical lesson to be learned from this demonstration is that the losses to time, while real, are inconsequential when compared to the losses due to disuse. A fit 70-year-old has lost the same amount of vitality as an unfit person many years younger. Fitness is a thirty- to forty-year age offset. This is why fitness for the young person is an option, but for the older person it is an imperative, as frailty and death loiter nearby.

As a long-distance runner, I identify easily that I am slower than thirty years ago. But turn me loose against an unfit 30-year-old, and I will leave him or her panting in my wake. Fitness compensates, even overcompensates, for age loss.

The terms "successful" and "usual" in connection with aging are used universally to denote the two trajectories of aging people. Usual aging is the standard, commonplace variety. Successful aging represents the theoretical ideal. Sure, there are changes due to aging that are real, measurable, and significant. But when contrasted to the changes due to disuse, they are unimportant to overall function. Usual aging is now quantified as a 2 percent decrement per year, whereas the successful aging rate is only ½ percent per year.

It is critical to observe that when the difference between usual and successful aging is examined over a short period of time—one year, for example—there is little apparent difference between the ideal and the standard. But when the 1½ percent yearly difference is multiplied over a number of decades, the differences are magnified. This observation comprises a central part of the optimism of this book.

How much am I as a human being really worth? If I were to take myself apart into my separate parts and try to sell myself on the open market, I wouldn't fetch very much. My hot air, my natural gas? Nothing. My body water? Probably less than a penny. As meat, as chemicals? Minimal. How about my blood? As a medical intern, I used to sell my blood to the blood bank to help augment my salary. The transplant business emerges as a way to profit by my organs, but I haven't really decided if I have a spare one of anything right now. The point is that none of us is worth very much by virtue of what we are. We achieve value by what we do. I am mortal and not physically worth much, but what I do is immortal and invaluable. The same is true for you.

My present body is a byproduct of my parents' romance, but more particularly my previous 65 years. My subsequent being is a product of its prior years, but more importantly, it is the product of the interplay of my hardware—molecules—with their present and future environment. They are diminished by the effects of time and injury. They are bettered by the effects of experience.

The resilience, the magnificent competence of our bodies is a full-blown glory if we maintain those bodies' potential, no matter our age. If we abdicate this potential to indolence either through ignorance or neglect, we deserve the lives we live. But if we have the guts and smarts to understand *how* we got this way, then the dare to be 100 becomes an achievable goal.

Remember this: If who you are is what you do, when you don't you aren't.

Chapter 3

Life Involvement

If the *when* of life is 100, the *what* of life is responsible choice, and the *how* is interactive (modeling of our possibilities), this is the smarts. It is the first part of the contract for 100 years. What remains is the guts, the *why*, the search for significance.

What makes a life significant? There scarcely could be a more important question. To tease out the anatomy of significance, certain features seem inevitable. Significance relates to need. It is generally social in nature. A life can't be significant in isolation. Further, significance has a time dimension. It is not just a passing item. Significance, too, implies an ordering of uncertainty and complexity. Fragmentation and disorder are not conducive to significance. Lastly, significance demands validation and gratification to be real.

Just as a home is more than walls, windows, and furniture, so, too, is life much more than bones and sinews and arteries, and even more than brain cells. Any full life is closely joined with other domains of human existence. The *why*, the guts, and the significance of life find opportunity in engagement, sex, flow, creativity, and wisdom.

"Successful and usual" are the two buzz terms used by

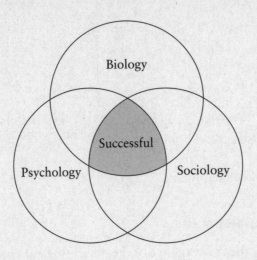

FIG. 5. Successful Aging.

most aging experts to denote the dominant trajectories of late life. Separating "usual" from "successful" means that a few old people don't seem to show the changes that most do. Some old folks have good memories, or good kidney function, or are still strong, when most aren't. Some are successful, but most are usual and failing. But, as I've mentioned before, aging well requires stamina and effort. Successful old age often consists of the ability to play a bad hand well.

In my view, successful means the ideal. But successful, ideal aging is not just biology. It is actually the intersection of the three basic domains of biology, psychology, and sociology—the three fundamental components of humanness.

Successful aging, successful life, occurs at the intersection of the three. Being bodily healthy, with a poor psychological or sociological domain, really is an empty bargain—and so it is with the other two combinations of these three vital components of successful aging.

You must be sound of body, mind, and social environment if you are to live and age ideally.

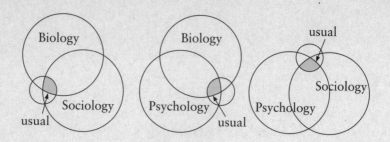

FIG. 6. Nonoptimal Aging.

ENGAGEMENT

Attitude is the convergence of the psychological and sociological domains of life, the A in DARE. It is the coming together of your mental competence, knowledge, and behavior with the social world in which you live.

The dominant theory in the psychology of aging is the theory of disengagement, first described over thirty years ago by Cumming and Henry in their book *Growing Old*. This theory holds that as a person ages he or she gradually loosens their bonds with the environment. They write and receive fewer letters, they go to fewer meetings, belong to fewer organizations, make and receive fewer phone calls, use their cars less, subscribe to fewer newspapers and magazines, have less to do with their family, and make love less often. They touch and are touched less. The older person falls away from the environment, and as a consequence the environment falls away from him or her. Risk taking diminishes. The older the person becomes, the less involved they become. The theory holds that many of these changes are natural, inevitable, and even desirable. Attendees of the conference of the South Carolina Commission on Aging were asked what they considered the main advantage was in growing older. The most common answer was less responsibility. The withdrawal motif is fed by social cues, health events, and institutional practice. The "empty nest syndrome" leads to the implication that life's main biological work is done, and the death of a spouse is a stern signal. Just as influential, retirement inevitably conveys a major sense of life passage for many.

The notion of disengagement involves more than just the external events of growing older; it involves the personal reactions to disengagement cues. Such isolation leads to vulnerability. Construction workers who are out of work and in poor financial straits suffer from risks to their health. Similarly, bereavement is always a dangerous time. It seems that while stress itself may not be so bad, it is lonely stress that causes real trouble.

In an effort to determine whether disengagement in older people is a matter of fate or choice, Stanford psychologist Laura Carstensen and her colleague Barbara Fredrickson at UC Berkeley devised an ingenious experiment. They first surveyed a healthy group of 240 community residents, 60 of whom were over 70 years of age. They assessed their degree of "engagement." Then they surveyed 120 gay men. The healthy gay men were found to be at least as engaged socially as the control straight subjects until they became HIV positive, at which point they pulled back and withdrew substantially from active life. Then Carstensen and Fredrickson assessed the subjects who were actually sick with AIDS and found that they were withered, withdrawn, and isolated. They had disengaged totally—not because they were old, but because they were getting ready to die. Therefore, disengagement was shown not to be an inevitable accompaniment of aging, but rather an act of will in anticipation of death.

What if a person disengages at age 65, with thirty-five more potential years of life out ahead? What if the wrong signals are sent and heard? What if "it isn't time yet"? Disengagement is not fate, it is choice. It is not inevitable and dependent on time. It can be reworked. You don't disengage because you are old. You become old because you disengage.

Only one quarter of those over the age of 75 still exhibit "high" social activity. Therefore, when a psychological profile of older people is carefully analyzed, it is found that a large number have disengaged. Still, many have not. Most are usual agers, while some are successful. Disengagement is to the psychological and sociological story as disuse is to the biological story.

My main point here is that both disuse and disengagement are preventable and reversible. As Laura Carstensen writes, "Beliefs about the irreversibility of psychological problems in the old are clearly untenable. The elderly are not, as a whole, a psychologically fragile group. It is an illusion that irremediable psychological deterioration is the modal course of old age."

In other words, disengagement is not and should not be a natural sidenote to aging. Psychological withdrawal is clearly a step in the wrong direction, just as remaining engaged in all that each day offers is clearly a leap in the right one.

SEX MATTERS

It is exactly at the same point of intersection of the three domains of successful being and aging where sexuality resides. Successful sexuality implies the active and robust participation of each of the three. Is such a coincidence merely haphazard, or do successful aging and successful sexuality share other features?

Sexuality is a point on the continuum of social relationships. The human is a social animal, engaged in relationships across a broad range of intensity, starting from the casual contacts with the postman or grocery clerk and extending next to broadly ranging, more committed states of friendship. At the high end of friendships are relationships in which sexual intimacy is a major bond. I maintain that physical health is directly tied to social health. It follows, then, that I should come to the conclusion that sex matters. Any survey taken to explore this assertion would end up with a unanimous agreement, particularly among younger people. As a teenager my recollection is that I spent 90 percent of unoccupied mind time fantasizing about sex. But sex shouldn't be confined to the first part of life. Is sex after 50 an unnatural act, a vestigial remnant of no biological value, or is it an integral and shaping part of the increasingly large part of our life spent after reproduction is over? For the rest of nature, sex is a purely reproductive event. But for humans, sex is recreational, as much as it is procreative, if not more so. We humans have uniquely harnessed it, like fire, for other purposes. Anthropologists teach us that continuous sexual receptivity was a technique evolved to keep the male close to home. In nature, sex and life and death are closely linked. Animals go to extraordinary lengths to position themselves to guarantee, or at least provide advantage for, their reproductive success, including individual sacrifice for the perpetuation of the species.

We exhibit no such life-endangering urgency in our reproductive pattern, or do we? Maybe the real reason men die around age 75 is not heart attacks or stroke, but because around age 65 they retire and—about the same time—start to lose their potency. As a result they disengage. Women clearly survive the loss of their ovaries, but can men survive the loss of their potency? They enter their 70s without the affirmation of who they are—their dominant roles in life apparently faded. Uselessness and impotency rule, and disengagement beckons as the logical strategy. In all other dimensions of their male lives they may be successful, but if their productive and sexual capacities are dimmed, their job descriptions constrict.

It is time to die, their economic and biological roles are ended, so why fight it? Hemingway, shortly before putting a shotgun in his mouth, said, "What the hell? What does a man care about? Staying healthy, working good. Eating and drinking with his friends, enjoying himself in bed. I haven't any of these—do you understand, goddam it? None of them!"

Of course, this is a radical proposition; but nonetheless it makes sense.

In a series on sex and aging, my colleagues and I found first that the group, average age 67, was a sexy group, sexier than we would have expected, and other previous surveys have shown the same. 53 percent of the men under 70 reported having sex at least once a week, as did 33 percent of those over 70. The corresponding figures for the women were 51 percent and 33 percent for the under- and over-70 groups, respectively. We figured that this represented the "usual pattern." However, when we asked how frequently they would like to have sex, 98 percent of the men under 70 desired sex once a week or more (66 percent desired two or more times per week), and the over-70 figures were virtually the same. Similar findings accompanied the women's trial. What is interesting about the results of this survey is that figures representing the desired rate of sex are almost identical to the reported sexual activity of ten years earlier.

These results indicated to us that these people in their late sixties and beyond had a major interest and involvement with the sexual components of their being. It was clearly a major quality-of-life determinant. Beyond that, they wished for more. At issue, too, were the two issues that separated our attendees from having the sexual lives they desired. For the men, the issue was impotence, but for the women it was opportunity. It seems that if we are to sustain life quality at its best level as we reach toward 100, both of these issues must be addressed.

First the men. Until recently, impotence was thought to be largely psychological in origin. Now this opinion has shifted totally as science identifies the mechanics of having an erection and what can go wrong with the apparatus. How the penis fills with blood is known in minute detail. The process follows a series of connected steps. Early in life these steps are in grand order, but with the passage of time increased amounts of collagen accumulate in the penis, making erections less sturdy. We now know that the feature that delays the deposit of collagen is blood flow. In other words, erections are good for erections. Unlike manmade machinery, in which a high degree of usage wears out the parts, for human machinery the opposite is true. Use it or lose it. Ill health, medication usage, and lack of a congenial partner are all negative conditions for the aging man. Fortunately, they can be counteracted.

And there is even more good news for us guys. The new knowledge about the process of developing an erection leads to the likelihood of drug compounds that will limit the deposits of collagen in the penis, thereby giving bright prospects of maintaining potency until advanced age.

And what about women? First, they are at a numerical disadvantage. We men simply must do a better job at living longer, and thereby participating in the intimacies of our mates as long as we both shall live. Various experts report that women's interest and capacity for sexual fulfillment do not diminish, until advanced old age, provided there is opportunity available. Clearly we need more information and broader avenues of communication. As we learn and talk more, old stigmas about sexual activity over 70 will erode and hopefully vanish.

Like other components of successful aging, sex must be open and embraced. Sex cannot be secret and successful at the same time. It needs permission and encouragement, and it particularly needs communication, which is finally what sex is all about in the first place. After all, sex is transmission of genetic, psychological, and spiritual energy. Like jogging, sex is preventive medicine. It makes you feel good and cuts down on health expenses.

GO FOR THE FLOW

Just as the Lonesome Cypress changes its whole shape in life to conform to the westerly winds, our social laws are impacted by the environments in which we live. At some times we feel we are in charge, operating at top efficiency, confident, successful, cruising. At other times, we feel out of sync, inept, down, inefficient, useless. Sometimes we are beached. Other times we are in flow. The entire domain of flow existence has been the life work of University of Chicago psychologist Mihaly Csikszentmihaly. He studies flow like I study blood pressure. Flow exists in all of us at some time, but for most it is rare. Only for a few is it fairly common. Flow is the state of being between stress and boredom. It is being in the zone of intense gratification, timelessness, and effortlessness. It is peak, mastery, ecstasy. It is total involvement with life.

Flow is also rare. You are in maximum flow no more than 1 percent of the time, but that is the moment of transcendence. If a task is too hard, you tend to lose heart; if it is too easy, you become bored. But when the conditions are right, and the effort is made, peak flow is the result. The other mundane issues of the world melt away in the recognition of accomplishment.

Csikszentmihaly found that we achieve flow when we are working at a challenging mental or physical task. In measured experiments, it's been determined that flow occurs mostly at work, much less during leisure. These experiments show that 54 percent of work time is spent in some degree of flow, 16 percent in boredom. At leisure, however, the reverse is true. You are in flow only 18 percent of the time, while 50 percent is dull and apathetic. Despite this clear distinction, many judge the leisure part of their lives as pleasurable. This observation, repeatedly confirmed, is called the paradox of work, which is specific to humans.

Perhaps evolution has selected humans on a flow quotient. We survive and flourish because we seem to spend more energy, and we are in turn rewarded for the expenditure. As a result, we achieve more reproductive success, which is nature's justification and reward for flow. Work releases adrenalin, which pumps out endorphins, which produce flow.

The resemblance of the processes involved in the products of flow experience bear striking similarity to growth activities in nature. A branch or a leg reacts to challenge by internalizing the energy it receives, repackaging it and then using the energy to do its work and to reconfigure itself to be more responsive to the challenge. The tissue resonates with its environment. It is in flow.

Not only is flow demonstrated to be that state of endeavor when we achieve the highest degree of integration with our work, it also represents that characteristic we find to be most admirable in others who triumph against great odds: the Helen Kellers, the little Davids, the Jack-and-the-beanstalks who are our heroes and heroines.

Flow is not just an instant. It represents a period of time. The more time we are in flow, the higher quality our lives will have. A young child appears to be in flow a great proportion of the time, but as we immerse ourselves in the adult business of living, barriers to flow emerge. Buckminster Fuller observed, "Everyone is born a genius, but the process of living degeniuses them." The losses of late life pose heightened dangers to the achieving of flow.

To maintain the opportunity for flow across a lifespan, you need guts and smarts—the smarts to identify the multiple sources of potential conflict with flow, and the guts for the energy and courage to offset the tendencies toward disengagement. Engagement is flow. Flow is engagement. If old age means disengagement, then flow has no chance. But if you keep the gears meshed and the motor running smoothly, you can sustain flow throughout your life.

The older years bring more freedom (which is flow conducive) and hopefully more perspective (which is also flow conducive). So during those years, flow doesn't have to decline. It can flow uphill—with guts and smarts to propel it. In fact, older people should have an advantage in this regard. Their repertoire of talents is greater. Their ability to distinguish what matters from what doesn't is greater, so that focus is greater. They're less self-conscious, and since self-consciousness is incompatible with flow, they have another advantage. I can't wait to grow older so I can have more flow.

CREATIVITY

The area of human creativity is a topic of great fascination. What made Mozart or Picasso or John Lennon so creative? What sets these people, whose work has done so much to enrich all of our lives, apart from the rest of us?

Creativity, be it artistic, personal, or scientific, has been said to consist of four phases—saturation, incubation, illumination, and validation. Saturation implies that the brain is filled to overflowing with all aspects of a topic. As a result of this phase, the multiple forms of the topic are free to roam in the brain circuitry, incubating—passing from right brain to left brain and back again, exposing new combinations and configurations. Then, wham! Illumination occurs as the spark strikes and the new circuit is created—a new sense, a new order, a new thought. The birth of a new idea represents ultimate flow.

This new idea, although seemingly creative, must first be validated. Drug and alcohol stupors conjure new patterns, but they are not relevant or confirmable. Without validation and relevance, creativity doesn't count. The laws of natural selection assert that only that new piece of matter which makes sense to the previous arrangements in nature should and will survive. For that reason, creativity demands validation and acceptance.

So creativity has four stages—saturation, incubation, illumination, and validation. As there is no single intelligence, there is no single creativity. Intelligence represents convergent thinking, in which facts are gathered and bundled. Creativity, on the other hand, represents divergent thinking. Instead of facts being joined by logic, they are rubbed together to form a new usually unexpected concept. Albert Szent-Gyorgy's memorable phrase about creativity is "to see what all have seen but think what none has thought." Intelligence and creativity are not synonymous. Often smart people aren't creative, and the most creative people aren't often those with huge intellects, although educator Howard Gardner feels that in order to have baseline smarts on which to draw, the creative individual must have an IQ or IQs of at least 120.

Creativity is rarely if ever genetic in its origin. The prodigy is extremely unusual. Gardner's research further indicates that most major creative efforts require at least ten years of saturation and incubation before illumination—that "Eureka!" moment—is reached. It takes another ten years for the next breakthrough moment to occur. Further, creative people tend to be sequentially creative, which means one-shot creativity is rare. Childhood is often the period in which the "capital of creativity" is banked. Frequently, creative people display a greed for knowledge, a tendency for experimental thought in early life. In his youth, Einstein pondered "gritty" problems, despite being a generally inept student. Picasso, too, was a poor student. Creativity occurs not on demand, but as a spontaneous outpouring of pleasure, flow.

If you accept the general premise that creativity is generally learned, rather than conferred by fate, it would seem that creative capacity should increase over the lifetime. But in practice the opposite seems to be the case. As Einstein stated, "A person who has not made his great contribution to science before the age of 30 will never do so." In general, it is held that productivity is highest in the 35 to 39 age range. Poets and mathematicians peak earlier, historians and philosophers later. Yet an article in the *Washington Post* showed several graphs of the creative powers of poets, novelists, inventors, physicists, and astronomers. All fields showed maximum creative success before age 50, but a number indicated a late-life surge after age 70. Michelangelo's *Pietà* done at age 89 seems more adventurous than the one done at 25. Barbara McClintock won her Nobel prize in her 80s. Schweitzer at Lambarene, Holmes in the Supreme Court, both at 90, were still vitally involved in creative efforts.

It is logical to presume that the first two phases of creativity, saturation and incubation, have a longer time to operate as an individual ages. The observation that often a ten-year period is necessary to produce the creative instant seems to confirm that time is a critical component for creativity. It is the illumination step that appears to be lacking in older people. Could it be that disengagement is the hurdle that impairs this luminous moment? Or is it comfort, security, and conformity that are inhibitive? Creativity has uniqueness and idiosyncrasy as centerpieces. If there is nothing novel or discontinuous in one's life, there is no creativity.

The rigidity that contemporary society imposes on youthful creativity is lamentable. Anthropologist Desmond Morris marveled at how chimps and young children showed exquisite delight at their venturing efforts with paint and paper. They are in flow. However, when their boisterous exploration is rewarded by various clues of approval or disapproval, the explorative behavior slackens and the primal joy is suppressed. In other words, when the individual experiences self-consciousness, the flow of creativity is blocked, spontaneity is blunted.

If we extend this observation to the human lifespan, we understand how the structures and incentives surround us and fence us in. If we know what is over the next ridge, why go?

Conversely, Michelangelo at age 89 said, "Thank God I can still learn." Despite nine decades of life, his boundaries were not set; his creative energy still worked.

Creating order out of chaos requires energy—we learned that earlier in the chapters on growth. If aging is characterized by an energy ebb, then sustaining creativity becomes more difficult. For the randomness of the world to congeal into a new moment of significance, energy must be directed to catalyze this reaction. All of us need to sustain our creative energies as we age.

I would guess that if creativity is to be cherished as a life goal—one not to be contained merely in the first part of life—then we need to provide sparks, congenial opportunities, and incentives for older people to exploit their natural experience for creative gain. We need "opportunity structures" in which older people can find their sparks and tend them.

Old people seem to be less in the business of creating things as creating selves. Many testimonials by older persons contain the message that age brings the opportunity "to be me" for the first time. For many, aging means nurturing the contented self, more time, more freedom, less dependence on external approval. Given such definition, late-life creativity takes on new significance, as late life is the only time during which such a reconciliation and unification can take place. Providing that that sustaining energy persists, the later phase of life should be the time of greatest—not least—creativity, the last for which the first was made. As Longfellow wrote:

> For age is opportunity no less
> Than youth, though in another dress
> And as the evening twilight fades away
> The sky is filled with stars, invisible by day.

WISDOM

The splendor of human existence is ultimately dependent on the ability of our minds to extract significant messages from the world in which we live. The brain, of course, is the organ that receives the messages, processes them, and tries to figure out what the hell is going on. The better trained it is, the better your life will be.

Memory loss with age is a huge demerit. Alzheimer's disease is a sullen fact of life. Alzheimer's disease is lightning, not normal aging, and it must, and will be, gotten rid of. But for the majority of persons, those without Alzheimer's disease, the fear of memory loss remains. What's the story?

When an old person is tested, he or she can remember six items, a young person eight. There is a real and confirmable difference in memory skills between young and old. However, when the older person undergoes a period of memory training, he or she can recall thirty items. Train a young person, and he or she will recall forty items. Again, the advantage goes to the young, but what is the more significant difference—young and old or trained and untrained? In just such a fashion I reckon that as I finished the Boston marathon in four and one-half hours, I was at the back of the pack. All the youngsters have left me far in their wake, but what about the millions of untrained persons who weren't there at all, and couldn't beat my time if their lives depended on it? Sure, age matters, but training and use of it are far more important.

Wisdom has been accorded great honor since the Greeks. Plato placed it at the pinnacle of human virtues. In his book *Survival of the Wisest*, Jonas Salk stated that wisdom provides alternative options and pathways in which to understand the multiple complexities the Earth provides. Wisdom implies lack of rigidity and allows us to view life as a dynamic process.

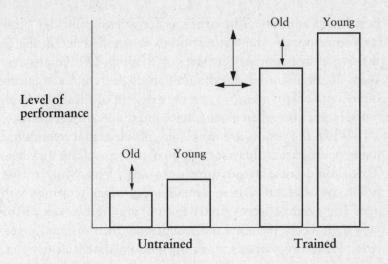

FIG. 7. Performance: Age vs. Training.

Paul Baltes is a superb psychologist interested in the mental profiles of older people. He has a particular interest in wisdom, which he defines as an expert knowledge system about life in general and good judgment about how to conduct oneself in the face of complex and uncertain circumstances. The five component parts of wisdom are factual knowledge, procedural knowledge, context knowledge, uncertainty knowledge, and relativeness knowledge. Each part has its own constituent aspects. For example, uncertainty knowledge would acknowledge that many situations have no ideal solution, that there is a balance between gains and losses, that the future is essentially unpredictable, and that fallback solutions are often the best. The criteria invoke the *what, when, how, where,* and *why* of life, as well as their infinite combinations.

Paul has devised a wisdom test that takes this theoretical framework into the real world. An intense, challenging social problem is posed to a test subject. Two favorite challenges: What if your 15-year-old daughter announces she wants to get married? How do you respond? Or What if your 40-year-old best friend announces he or she is considering suicide? How do you respond? The test responses are graded according to the five above component parts of wisdom. Do the answers show depth of knowledge of facts, strategies, contexts, uncertainty, and relativeness, or are they devoid of these rich contents, based instead on more fragile and diminished resources?

When the results are tabulated, it's clear that overall not many people are truly wise ever, no matter how long they live. This should come as no surprise to any of us. More to the point, over a lifetime, there is no falloff in wisdom ratings with age. The average seems pretty even overall. However, of the very high raters, most are old, confirming their original suspicion. Therefore, Baltes's work on wisdom shows clearly that old age can be a time of continued personal growth. As Joan Erikson, wife of Harvard psychologist Erik Erikson, wrote in an interview in the *New York Times*, "Not all old people are wise, but you don't get wise until you are old."

The view of the gains possible with age are seated in an acknowledgment of losses. An example cited by Paul Baltes involves Arthur Rubenstein, who related his own personal strategy as an aging pianist. First, he restricted his repertoire to fewer pieces. Second, he practiced them more often. Third, he intentionally slowed his playing before the parts of the piece that were rapid, so as to increase the impression of speed by contrast. Similarly, old typists have been shown that they can retain typing speed by anticipating upcoming words. Such anticipation can compensate for the decrease in neurological processing. Remember, aging does bring gains with the losses.

In summary, then, as we survey the "so what?" of growing old, we reexamine the elements of engagement, sex, flow, creativity, and wisdom. Victor Hugo wrote, "If you look in the eyes of the young you see flame. If you look in the eyes of the old you see light." In these domains we find the deeper essence of being alive. Common features of aging are energy, directedness, and time. These are the features of growth.

Figure 8 is borrowed from a depiction conceived by Marian Diamond, a scientist whose research involves brain enrichment. In it is represented how features of psychological supremacy are translated into biological form, and vice versa. When a brain cell is at its most rudimentary, it has a few small twigs or branches (dendrites). These early outcrops found in youth are concerned with the basic needs of comfort and security. As development proceeds, other competences emerge, as more experience yields more complex possibilities. With maximum growth engagement, flow, creativity, and wisdom are exhibited, as the brain cell is at its full expression. It becomes connected and competent.

It is in age when this flowering has its best opportunity, if we only have the guts and smarts to encourage it. A broad

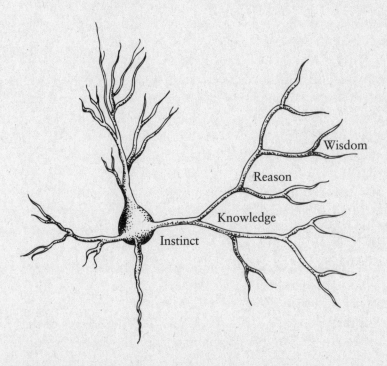

FIG. 8. Simplified diagram of brain cell development.

survey of the psychological and social aspects of successful aging reveals a recurrent theme. Attitude follows the same dynamic as the body—use it or lose it. When a leg is casted, it withers. When you disengage, you wither emotionally, intellectually, and socially, with a cascade of negative events sure to follow. Conversely, if you exercise a withered leg, it renews its strength and purpose. In reengaging, you achieve flow, enable creativity, and allow wisdom and meaning to emerge. Time is the catalyst, but without continued involvement, a lifetime alone is insufficient. Time and energy are the combustion mix that makes matter matter. In other words, sustaining involvement over the lifespan makes for successful aging. Anything less is merely usual.

Chapter 4

The Roots of 100

We tend to think of something old as something in the past. But really, "old" refers to the future. What the future holds for us, in other words, is old age. If old is the future, what will it look like? Let's look at the centenarians. As Socrates wrote, "It is good that we should ask the old who have gone along a road we must all travel in our turn the nature of that road."

What is a centenarian? What is so special about them that we should hitch our wagons to their star? When asked how it felt to be 100, one centenarian replied, "I don't know. I've never been 100 before." Tongue in cheek, George Burns has said, "If you live to the age of 100 you have it made, because very few people die past the age of 100." Is 100 just a numerical artifact that has no biological importance—a curiosity—or is there a deeper significance to living a century? To answer these questions, let's look at the data. Let's look at who centenarians are, what they have done, and where they have come from.

Today's centenarians were born in the 1890s, when Grover Cleveland and McKinley were president. There were forty-four states. The American population was 63 million. Average life expectancy was 45 years. Seventy-five percent lived in poverty. Ten percent had a high-school education. Horse and buggies, covered wagons, outdoor plumbing, gold in the Alaska Klondike, Indian treaties, Spanish-American War, first pro football game in Latrobe, Pennsylvania. Bloomers, fedoras, long swimming suits. Babe Ruth was born, Adolph Hitler and Charlie Chaplin were little boys. Queen Victoria. First Nobel Prize. *La Bohème* premieres. World population 1.6 billion. First modern Olympic games in Athens. No radio, movies, TV. No income tax. First telephone, first photos. Kitty Hawk was twenty years in the future.

In my home town Senator Leland Stanford bought 740 acres with one barn and three houses for $300,000 and named it Palo Alto. In 1894 Palo Alto was incorporated by a vote of 88 to 21. In 1885 there was a general store, a blacksmith shanty, a wood yard, several livery stables, and a carriage painting shop. The pride was two horse-drawn fire wagons for the volunteer fire company. Justice was administered by Constable Roger Spalding, known as "Old Sleuth." A six-room house sold for less than $2,000. In 1895 there were sixteen births, one death and five weddings reported. Electricity came in 1896. By 1899 there were three churches. The WCTU made life tough for the saloons.

The *Palo Alto Times* of 1895, under the headline "May the Gods Preserve Us," editorialized: "We hoped we might escape, but we have caught it. A women's suffrage club is to be permanently organized Saturday afternoon. We suppose we may pray for grace and be reconciled in the thought that as colic, mumps, and measles are common to childhood so every new town shows infantile mental disease. Fathers, husbands, sons, and brothers should observe a strict quarantine in this crisis, and we might experience only a light attack of this epidemic."

I have several patients who were alive then and still are. Palo Alto is a city now of 56,000 with no horse and buggies, a few barns, but property worth billions of dollars. As my city celebrates its 100th birthday the centenarians are the center-piece. Two patients are children of Al Wherry, an original resident who died recently, aged 103. Al rode in the honored car of our town's centennial celebration. Jane Shurr, public information officer at the National Institute on Aging, terms the centenarians a "living national treasure," caretakers of tradition and culture. Their personal stories are as much of our nation's history as are the newspaper headlines. Yet their work and experiences are seldom recorded. In 1987 President Reagan proclaimed July first National Centenarian's Day. Senator Claude Pepper felt that living to be 100 was the supreme personal privilege.

The centenarians are the most rapidly growing segment of the American population, that is clear, but their numbers are unclear. The reason for this is that, until relatively re-cently, record keeping was pretty scattered. Not until 1933, when Texas signed on as the last state, was the Federal Death Registry fully complete. American birth and death records are supplemented more recently by information provided by the Social Security Administration and Medicare. But these, too, have had their problems. Some recalculations have been necessary because of honest and not-so-honest mistakes made in some claims and reports. Other countries are even more retarded in their vital statistics about age. As a result, age figures are often dependent on church records, Bibles, and memory. In my travels, I spend as much time as far away as I can get. There I find the people to be amazingly uninter-ested in birthdays or even age. It is not how old that counts, it is what you can do. The calendar is meaningless to the Kalahari Bushmen. What matters for them is only whether they are frail. Not until then, regardless of age, do they consider themselves "old."

The most-publicized longevity reports concerned a study by Dr. Alex Leaf, formerly chief of medicine at Massachusetts General Hospital, and one of America's most highly regarded physicians. In 1971 he traveled to Hunza, the Caucasus, and Villcamba, Ecuador, to search out the mythic Shangri-Las of aging. He reported his findings in the *National Geographic* in January 1973 and in the medical journal *Hospital Practice* later that year. The appeal of the articles was enormous. Here was the sought-for evidence that there existed somewhere over the rainbow places where life was so sweet that people could live on and on unstressed by the ravages of civilization. Dr. Leaf reported on and pictured Shiral Mislimov, said to have been born in 1805, listening to a transistor radio. He still rode horseback and told of his 102-year marriage to his wife, who was only 120. Various calculations led Dr. Leaf to conclude that another individual, Khfaf Lasuria, was either 134 or 144 or 138 or 132 or 131. No records remained, but she remembered how old she was on different occasions. Everyone in that area expects to live to be 100. Unfortunately, when other scholars returned to these areas to confirm ages, they concluded that "There is no convincing proof that anyone has lived more than 120 years."

The oldest current living person is listed in *The Guinness Book of World Records* as Jeane Louise Calment of Arles, France. Her birth certificate is dated February 21, 1875. She recalls having sold colored pencils to Van Gogh when she was 14. "He was ugly as sin, was hot tempered, a grumbler, and smelled of alcohol." Several years ago she gave up her two cigarettes a day and her port, but she still loves chocolate. Deaf and nearly blind from cataracts that she refuses to have fixed, she moves around by wheelchair—the result of a hip fracture suffered in a fall at age 115. She lived alone in a second-story apartment with no elevator and no hot water service until the age of 110, when the plumbing froze and she decided to move to a nursing home. She had no major illnesses before then. Her wit is clearly intact. "I have only one wrinkle, and I am sitting on it," she joked. At almost 119, Madame Calment was the subject of an in-depth psychological interview, complete with a brain CT scan. Her performance on tests of verbal memory and language fluency were equivalent to that of people forty years younger, and her cognitive function was actually found to improve over a six-month observation period. She still rode her bike until age 115 and still wears rouge. She remarked, "I waited 110 years to become famous, and I intend to enjoy it as long as possible." But, when asked what kind of future she expected, she replied, "A very short one." In their coverage of her birthday, the *Washington Post* told of a real-estate practice in her part of the world called *viager*. This verb describes the practice of assuming the home mortgage payment of an old person. Not until the person dies can the mortgage payor claim the house. Usually this works out well for the payor, but not in the case of Jeane Calment. Thirty years ago a local notary public made a terrible real-estate deal: He bought her house. Each year she sends him a note that reads, "Excuse me if I'm still alive, but my parents didn't raise shoddy goods." On Christmas Day in 1995 the notary died, having paid out over 40 years four times what the house is worth. Meanwhile, Madame Jeane Calment keeps on ticking.

Closer to home, centenarians in American are estimated at 22 per 100,000 population. The oldest living American is thought to be Minnie Kolb, born March 7, 1879. One hundred years ago, the chance of a baby living to be 100 was 1 in 500; now it is 1 in 80 and getting better. If you want to move to a state where you will have the best chances, go to Hawaii, where 2 percent of the population will reach 100. Minnesota and South Dakota are close behind. If you don't care much about being 100, move to Washington, D.C., or Alaska, where your chances of making 100 are about half as good. The 1980 American census initially reported 32,000 centenarians, but a recalculation reduced this by half. The error was reportedly due to "processing and respondent error."

Our last census, in 1990, counted 36,808 American centenarians. Based on this and further projections, it is estimated the number will grow to 100,000 by 2000, and one million by 2050, you and I among them. If we simply follow the commonsense health practices that we already recognize as beneficial, we will not be talking about 2 or 4 or 8 percent living to 100, but the majority of the population. Talk about a mega-trend!

AGE ARCHIVES

Someone observed that there are lots of books about old cars, old churches, old painting, and old furniture, but very few about old people. True. UCLA gerontologist Roy Walford did discover one book, written by James Easton in 1799—*Human Longevity Recording the Name, Age, Place of Residence and Year of the Decease of 1712 Persons who Attained a Century and Upwards from* A.D. *66 to 1799, Comprising a Period of 1733 with Anecdotes of the Most Remarkable*—and in the last decade or so there have been several books published about centenarians from different perspectives. These reveal an increasingly confident picture of what 100 years of living looks like. The most noted of these is the Delaney sisters' *Having Our Say* published in 1993, which played on Broadway as a smash hit. It is the life history of two fine women, daughters of a man born as a slave but who eventually became the first black Episcopal bishop. The story is one of grit and determination. Bessie Delaney (the younger one of the Delaney sisters) passed away recently at the age of 104, but her portrait of her life offers inspiration and poignancy to the journeys of the rest of us.

As Viktor Frankl commented, "Life achieves meaning when it serves as an example to others." As we look into the lives of these centenarians we see ourselves 30 or 50 or 70 years from now.

LIVES TO CHERISH

Tales of lives fully lived reveal much to those of us who will follow. They include the story of Clyde Ice of Spearfish, South Dakota, who flew in a small airplane on his 100th birthday. After having participated in the South Dakota centennial celebration, he got to bed at 3:30 A.M. that special day and arose at 8:00 A.M. the next morning for the Clyde Ice Day at the Reno Air Show, which for him was highlighted by meeting President Bush. He remarked, "The biggest problem I have is that my landing gear is worn out, and I can't get around like I used to. The rest of me is just as good as twenty years ago."

Two recent obituaries taught us much about the richness made possible by living long lives. Rose Kennedy, 1891 to 1995, lived a life of incredible texture. A record of her life experience would fill libraries, and, indeed, innumerable volumes on the personal and political history of the Kennedys have been written. And playwright/producer George Abbott, age 107, died January 31, 1995. Of Abbott, George Milstein of the *New York Times* wrote in 1954, "On the basis of sheer frightening volume alone an easily defensible argument can be drummed up that no living individual, or possibly ever alive, has contributed more to Broadway than George Abbott." In 1994 Abbott watched his own work *Damn Yankees* performed at the Marquis Theater, just as he had forty years earlier. As a testimony to the source of his longevity, his third wife, whom he married at age 96, said, "Work, work, work. That's what kept him going." In fact, he was working on a revision of the second act of *Pajama Game* when he died. In addition to his fully realized creative life, his legacy to millions of theatergoers was great competence and grace.

And there are, of course, many less celebrated centenarians whose stories are enlightening. Interviewed by the *New York Times* while driving his Cadillac in the fast lane on the Merritt Parkway, Eli Finn started classes at Fairfield University at age 100. One centenarian was pardoned on his 100th birthday for killing a neighbor with a branding iron after rustling a horse. John Gardner of Alagash Plantation, Maine, lived in the same house for 100 years. Mrs. Florence Doleph (1847–1949), was cited in the *London Times* for sliding down a banister on her 100th birthday. Beatrice Salmon Plant received her college degree from the University of Toronto when she was 100. At 97, Mieczyslaw Horszowski played a piano recital to a sold-out Carnegie Hall audience. *The New York Times* review called his playing "lustrous," "playful," and "poignant." Beatrice Wood, a 103 year-old-sculptor, asserted, "It's only the covering that grows old."

On an excursion to Baja California I visited an old Mexican who lived in El Cardonal, north of Cabo San Lucas. Pablo Geraldo was born sometime in September of 1887. His mother died at age 90, while his father, a fisherman, had died young. Pablo, who had seven children, and many grandchildren, had scarcely traveled out of his tiny village in his 106 years. He was married over 70 years. He never went to school, and could not read or write. He didn't smoke, but he did have an occasional tequila. His only medicine was a lime drink, which he took for his arthritis. Twenty years ago he had had a hernia repair, but otherwise was well until he fell two weeks before my visit and broke his hip. His vision and hearing and memory were excellent. He loved music. The priest visited regularly. I checked his pulse—65 beats per minute, strong and regular. He reported he was "very happy."

Shirley Potter bungee-jumped 210 feet in Alpine, California, to celebrate his 100th birthday. He lamented, however, that the subsequent publicity was "killing me." *Newsweek* of May 4, 1992, showed Claire Will taking dance classes at 100. Genevieve McDaniel, 102, taught aerobics. David Eldridge of St. Petersburg still umpired at 105. Otto Aster (1863–1966) at 103 was said to be America's oldest roller skater. Herman

Smith-Johansen cross-country skied five miles at age 100. Harlow Potter, 103, was the oldest of the 8,000 competitors in the 1995 Senior Sports Classic. He took up golf at age 92 and recently shot a 98.

Aside from providing inspirational centenarian stories, I'd like to offer some interesting longevity statistics: First, women tend to outlive men over the lifespan by a substantial margin. Male centenarians represent only 20 percent of the sample, but somewhat paradoxically, 40 percent of those over 105 are men. Further, examination of the ethnic origin of centenarians is revealing. Among the centenarians counted by the 1990 census, 237 were American Indian, Eskimo, or Aleut. Chief Red Cloud, a Sioux, was said to be born in the Oklahoma Territory in 1842, was married four times, fathered thirty-six children (his last at age 90), and died in 1962. Chief Tommy Thompson (1854–1959), leader of the Wyoming Indians, had this formula for longevity: "Don't drive an automobile, and eat lots of salmon." At 92 Chief Red Cloud of the Chickawas married Losette Cloud. At 100 he was struck by a car, broke both legs, recovered, and lived on to survive a bout of pneumonia at age 111.

Also of major note is the fact that, although African-Americans constitute only 12 percent of the general population, they represent 18 percent of the centenarians. This is in accord with the observation that, although black people are less likely to survive into old age than white people, when they do, they tend to outlive whites. Similarly, the male-female survivorship differential is lower in blacks than whites. Whereas over 40 percent of white centenarians are confined to an institution, only 13 percent of blacks are. My speculation on these curious findings is that survivorship has a lot to do with maintaining a social role, particularly within the family. I have often been impressed with how black people maintain a meaningful family participation—even to advanced ages.

Twenty-four percent of male centenarians are still married, whereas only 4 percent of female centenarians have a husband. One hundred men are recorded as having married after the age of 100, but only one woman. A centenarian couple was married for 84 years. Centenarians also get divorced. The above cited *National Geographic* article quotes a 100-year-old Azerbaijan, who "married my 7th wife 3 years before. My first 6 were all wonderful women but this present wife is an angry woman and I have aged at least 10 years since marrying her. If a man has a good and kind wife he can easily live 100 years." The article's author observed that old people with many children seemed to live the longest. Two of these prolific parents were baptized after 100. One centenarian had married nine times. Two children were the most frequent family size. Four families had six generations—great, great, great grandchildren. One centenarian had fifteen children after age 50. Seventy-eight percent of centenarians lived largely in one locale, 33 percent in one place all of life. Sixty percent were still living with another family member.

The important qualifier in any survey inquiring whether individuals want to live to 100 is health. Being sick and feeble for 100 years doesn't sound like a very good deal to anyone. An article in the January 1995 *Scientific American* by Thomas Perls entitled "The Oldest Old" explores the notion that very old people seem to be healthier than younger people, possibly as a result of their hardiness. Though some centenarians have been invalids for most of their life, the general health status of most centenarians is amazingly frisky. Thirty-one percent rate their health as excellent, 42 percent as good, 20 percent fair, 5 percent poor, and 2 percent very poor. Most don't have a family doctor, and many never saw a doctor. One said, "I see a doctor every 100 years." They think health, not dwelling on sickness and death. Foiling the doc is an issue of pride. Centenarians expect to live. Some think of illness as "a breathing spell." Emma Schott (1860–1960), of Washington, D.C., was kicked by a horse at age 8 and was told she wouldn't live, and she still lived to be 100. She commented, "The horse is dead, the doctor is dead, and I'm 100." Surgery is increasingly common and safe in those over 100. Thirty-one percent of centenarians manage all their own self-care. Eighty-four percent function well. Sixty-eight percent report arthritis. Seventy-two percent are mobile without canes or walker. Eight percent are in wheelchairs, 5 percent in beds.

In a study of social security enrollees, 56 out of 1,200 were in the hospital in the past year. Most report a good or excellent memory. An 109-year-old observed, "I don't occupy my mind with things that are unnecessary."

Vision was decreased in 29 percent, but 8 percent used no glasses. Only 4 percent were blind. Thirty percent had decreased hearing, which was judged to be more of a burden than decreased vision. Few lost taste or smell. Two-thirds had dentures. Charlie Smith, age 136 or 104 (depending on which source), used his teeth for "special" occasions. Otherwise, he kept them on his mantelpiece, like other decorations.

With regard to health, mobility and survival seem to be tightly linked. Ninety-one percent of male centenarians could walk, 85 percent of women. Seventy-five percent of men and 60 percent of women could still climb stairs. Next to work, walking was considered the best old-age prescription. Belle Boone Beard writes in *Centenarians: The New Generation,* "Nothing is more detrimental to the health and happiness of very old people than to deny them the privilege of walking."

Few cigarette smokers reach 100. In *Centenarians,* Belle Boone Beard cites a survey in which only 10 of 337 were cigarette smokers. Cigar or pipe smoking or tobacco chewing was more prevalent. Over 50 percent drank alcohol. Most ate breakfast, and 58 percent ate three meals and were lean, but a low-fat diet was not a habit they shared. As part of a centenarian study being conducted at the University of Georgia, Mary Ann Johnson surveyed the dietary habits of a number of centenarians. She found no vegetarians. Although meat was not highly preferred, bacon and sausage were common breakfast fare. Fifty-two percent took extra vitamins and minerals. Only calcium intake was found to be below the common RDAs, and 1,700 to 1,900 calories per day was the average daily intake. Overweight, although not unknown, was rare, and most Georgia centenarians drank coffee or tea regularly.

Of all the longevity prescriptions offered by the centenarians, work was number one. One said at 100 "you could do all you could at fifty, except that it takes longer." Belle Boon Beard cites another survey in *Centenarians* where 100 of 555 were still making money after 100. Some practiced law, some medicine; some were watchmakers. Dr. J. Reuben Branscomb, at age 106 in Fancy Gap, Virginia, in the Blue Ridge Mountains, reported that he had delivered over 2,500 babies, the last at age 100. Nearly every person living in a forty-mile radius was brought into the world by his gentle hands. In some families he had delivered three generations of babies. He finally gave up making house calls at age 100.

In general, centenarians disregard advice to take it easy. Pulitzer Prize winner John Netherland Heiskell (1872–1972), of Little Rock, Arkansas, was the oldest active newspaper editor in the U.S. Ed Hanau, 100, of St. Louis was still working at a manufacturing plant, having never missed a day of work in his life. As discussed earlier, work seems to be a biological necessity. Eighty-nine percent of centenarians report having worked hard during their lives. Only 10 out of 1,200 had "easy lives." Only those who disregard the advice to slow down lived to 100. Seven percent worked over 90 years, 92 percent worked over 60 years. Only 3½ percent retired at age 65. Seventy out of 1,200 men were still working for wages, and 219 of 1200 were still working past 100, predominantly in the house.

Centenarians are characterized by having realistic outlooks, efficiency in lifestyle, and lack of self-consciousness. They are socially adjustable, harmonious, frugal, flexible, optimistic, interested, humble, and patriotic. They are not afraid of death or of life. They show a quiet gusto, nonaggressive determination, a soft fortitude. They are positive, challenged, and useful. Their posture tends to reflect the feeling, "I don't worry about things over which I have no control."

These centenarians are our future. They are the rootstock onto which our lives are grafted. When they were born life was simpler, but for almost all it was also shorter. They are clearly durable, made out of "good dust." They maintained a good resonance with their world, and now they are old. They have aged successfully, productively, responsibly, usefully. They are 100 because they dared.

The centenarians of today are living two or three generations longer than the average life expectancy when they were born. Expectancy is easier now, and people reach 100 without a prearranged plan. The ones who reached 100 before us did so by fate. Now it is our opportunity to make it happen by choice.

Chapter 5

Gameplan for Life

When considering a trip, you will want to know how far you want to travel, where you want to go, when you want to leave, what route you will take, and how much it will cost. Life's journey implies the same sort of planning. You know, or should know, where you are now. Your destination is 100 healthy years. When you leave is now. The question is, How do you get from here to there?

Knowing how far the destination is allows you to make plans. Choice has replaced fate as the strategy. Choice implies using experience and other accumulated knowledge to show the way. Progress proceeds by little steps preceded by knowledge. These days we can organize and plan our lives with a high likelihood of accuracy. Life becomes self-fulfilling. We get what we set. In pursuit of understanding this idea of life planning, I believe a sports model helps. Life can be thought of as a game. Someone once said that life is the one race you win by finishing last. Life is a contest of skills held over time. It is a struggle. It can either be won or lost, and by big or little scores. Each of us will live our lives better if we have a gameplan.

In the school of life that I have been attending all my days,

Bortz U, one of my most stimulating, resourceful, and unexpected teachers has been Bill Walsh, former coach of the San Francisco 49ers and Stanford University. No one can sensibly question Bill's place in the pantheon of football coaches. There simply has never been anyone better. Much of the basic schemes of coaches at all levels arose first as Xs and Os in Bill's cerebral cortex. A number of current major coaches were his assistants.

I first met Bill when I was asked to help take care of his dad through a long and sad terminal illness. I well recall being with Bill in Washington in 1981 just after the 49ers had demolished the Redskins in a night game. The drama and thrill of this gaudy victory left me giddy, but Bill was solemn and distracted as he remembered his dad's inglorious decline.

I have now had the great fun to watch Walsh teams in three situations—first at Stanford, then with the 49ers, and then again back at Stanford. In each domain Walsh football has not only been great fun to watch, but the carefully studied design and preparation for each play, for each game, and for each season has provided life lessons of tremendous value.

The Walsh program leaves little to chance—even the most improbable game situation is prepared for in advance. His approach leads to extension by analogy to the game of life. Bill's sense of organization and preparation is the antithesis of the playground game, in which the kids' huddle strategy consists of "everybody out for a long one." This scattershot strategy rarely works, and when it does it succeeds only because the defense is even more disorganized than the offense.

In each incarnation Walsh has brought a systematic approach to the game. One of his trademark tactics is to script the first twenty-five plays to be used in the game. This foreknowledge is clearly apparent in the crispness and confidence with which the teams assume the first offense. His players have practiced, rehearsed, anticipated, and visualized these plays in advance—the sense of preparation is evident. The defense guesses, but the Walsh teams know. This scripting allows the players to be in control—it relieves the uncertainties. Anxiety and stress often accompany the start of the game, but Walsh's 49ers particularly were masters at overcoming these conditions. Their strategy helped sort out the complexities of the first violent confrontation.

The jump-start component of the Walsh gameplan is well identified, but it is in late-game tactics that Bill's understanding of the game really stands out. No situation is so desperate, unexpected, or chaotic that advance planning has not anticipated it. Fate is allowed no role—every contingency is anticipated. 49ers quarterback Joe Montana's place in the Hall of Fame derives largely from the extraordinary record the 49ers had as a game or the half draws to a close. "The two-minute offense" was virtually defined by Walsh teams. I will never forget the last drive Joe executed in the 1989 Super Bowl, Bill's last game as 49ers coach. As tens of millions of eyes looked on, Montana took the 49ers the length of the field to victory.

From 1983 to 1988, the 49ers scored twenty-two touchdowns and twenty-one field goals in the last two minutes of the first half. This computes to a score in 41 percent of the opportunities. Similarly, they dominated at the end of the game as well, yielding many "miracle" finishes. But they weren't miracles. They were planned. They were scripted, just like the last act of a play.

If you left at halftime or at the end of the third quarter, you certainly missed the full glory. Early in my days of Walsh watching, I missed important parts of the strategy. The 49ers have had outstanding pass rushers, notably Fred Dean and Charles Haley. Their specific task was to make the life of the opposing quarterback as miserable as possible by harassment and intimidation. Curiously, Bill frequently held these specialists out of the action in the early quarters. I joined many fans in yelling for their presence early in the game. But Bill knew what it was all about. He reasoned that the pass rushers were particularly valuable at the end of the game. Just when the game was in doubt, the opponent was urgently trying to regroup and catch up, but they were also tired—exactly the situation Bill wanted. He wanted his troops fresh and fired up, to pressure and exploit the opposition at the last critical moments. In contrast, Joe Montana was being chased by opponents whose legs were leaden from being expended early in the game. The last minutes of the game almost always belonged to Bill's teams, because of the gameplan.

Occasionally a Walsh team fell behind early in the game. One year Stanford fell behind 22–0 to Georgia in the Bluebonnet Bowl game; however, they rallied to win 25–22. Similarly, Stanford trailed Notre Dame 18–0 early one game. Things looked very bleak. But Bill's teams had rehearsed for this scenario. They knew that the score that counts is not the one at halftime but at the final whistle. They came back and won. Such preparation led, too, to the 49ers coming back from a 35–3 halftime deficit to win 38–35 against the New Orleans Saints.

Not only do Walsh teams do well at the end of individual games, but they also perform superbly late in the season. Again, their success is no accident. Bill credits this extraordinary success in December games to a strategy of avoiding debilitating harsh practices early in the season. Other teams, in their efforts to stay sharp and tough for the long grind, maintain vigorous practice scheduled over the six-month season, leading almost inevitably to crucial injuries during practice and game times, at just the worst times. Bill reasoned differently. "It's a long season. We will conserve our energies for the last part. We want to be tough at the end and not just early and in the middle of the season." Right, wonderful, imperative reasoning—why didn't somebody else think of that?

Bill disdains the quick fix, the temporary advantage. He insists on the gameplan. We were in his box at Candlestick

Park in 1988 on the occasion of the amazing hair-raising scramble that quarterback Steve Young pulled off late against the Minnesota Vikings to win the game. Steve bounced off nearly every Viking on his run to the end zone, finishing off with an exhausted, headlong dive over the goal line. This run made all highlight films, but it upset Bill a lot. After the game, he reflected only on the fact that improvisation is not the way to win in the long run. One touchdown doesn't make the season. You don't score each time the center snaps the ball, so it is with the ensemble of orderly plays that prevails over the long haul. Delay gratification.

Treating Vince Lombardi's "winning is everything" approach circumspectly, Bill has developed amazing insights into the time dimensions of the game through his own steady development as a coach. He played the role of assistant much longer than most coaches. He was disappointed over and over by his lack of promotion to head coach, but when it happened, a series of successes followed. He placed emphasis on treating the second-team players as if they are starters, so they could step in if a starter was hurt.

Today, Bill still prepares for bad weather, unexpected penalties, injuries, crowd noise, and so on, and he always takes pride in the high success rate of his teams when playing on the opponents' turf. His planning process was even recognized by a major article in the 1993 *Harvard Business Review,* which noted Bill's ability to sublimate the needs of his own ego to the success of his team. A younger coach would not have such perspective.

Planning allows overcoming of superior talent. The 1981 Super Bowl victory was achieved not only with a low payroll, but with clearly inferior talent. Bill estimates that 85 to 90 percent of success is in the preparation, 10 to 15 percent in talent.

In this regard, a recent *New York Times* report on peak performance noted that world-class violinists practice twice as much as nationally acclaimed violinists, who practice twice as much as local violinists. Such a relationship holds for chess masters as well. Directed effort, planning, and practice makes the performance; the performance makes the person. In his book *The Mind's Sky,* Timothy Ferris of UC Berkeley has a chapter titled "Joe Montana's Prefrontal Cortex." Ferris estimates that the development of a portion of Joe's brain associated with throwing the fifteen-yard down-and-out pass is extraordinarily developed. In the days before the last of Bill's Super Bowls, I watched Steve Young throw sideline passes over and over to receiver Jerry Rice long after the others had gone to the dressing room. Similarly, Marian Diamond showed that the association and computation part of Einstein's brain was hypertrophied, like a weight lifter's biceps.

Another of my professors at Bortz U was Paul Spangler. I first met Paul sixteen years ago at a track meet. He was only 80 then. Paul became a surgeon and was surgeon in chief at Pearl Harbor when the Japanese attacked; later he served with Project Hope. During these middle years, he was not involved in fitness. He had no life gameplan, even though he'd been on the University of Oregon track team as an undergraduate. At age 54 he was fat, stressed, and out of shape. Then Paul decided it was time to change. He started to run again. He lost thirty pounds and embarked on a totally new career. He became a model for fitness. He became a widely sought after speaker on the health benefits of physical exercise, and he began to compete—boy, did he compete—locally, nationally, and internationally. Paul was always there in his running shoes and blue blazer, which carried the emblem of adviser to the President's Council on Physical Fitness and Sport. He focused the remainder of his life to being an exemplar of the healthy life.

Late in his career Paul was often the only competitor in his age group, say 90 to 95. In Australia, in 1992, he won six gold medals for running and swimming, and altogether he probably held more gold medals than anyone since Nero. The day before he was to run a race, I asked him what his likely time was going to be. He replied, "I really don't know, but whatever it is will be a world record."

Paul had hoped to be the first centenarian to run a marathon. The oldest person so far to achieve this goal was a 98-year-old Greek. Paul finished the New York Marathon at age 92 and had on his schedule to do it again in November 1999, at age 100. Unfortunately, he died last April, at age 95, while running at 5:30 A.M. near his home in San Luis Obispo.

I had examined him a few weeks before. He had poor balance and had fallen and broken two ribs. He was a little anemic, and his heart skipped, but his mind and spirit were razor sharp. All of us who knew and loved Paul were shocked by his death. His slow, stately pace had been a metronome by which we all could hear the tempo. He set his goal and damn near made it, but what a way to go!

I am a proud member of the Fifty Plus Fitness Association. We are a growing organization of about 2,000 members nationwide who are bonded in the effort to demonstrate the value of a physically active lifestyle as we age. We are all participants in a number of research projects, the most notable of which is led by Dr. Ralph Paffenbarger, the eminent epidemiologist who leads the famous Harvard Alumni study. A recent survey of our membership, which was picked up by Jane Brody for the *New York Times* health column, showed that our members had one quarter the expected mortality and disability as others our age. Our newsletter is a collection of different reports from the scientific literature and from our members that show the essential nature of fitness in our later years. Once a year we hold our annual bash. It involves lectures, workshops, demonstrations, an awards banquet, and a walk, bike ride, and run that finishes in the Stanford Stadium. You must be over 50 to participate, however. (Youngsters must delay their gratification!) This year fifteen people over 80 took part in the race.

Also at our meeting this year was Ron Clarke from Australia. Ron, now 58, was one of the greatest runners of all time. Ron was a spectacular guest, participating in every part of our weekend. He even ran our race. Now all of us there can say, "I ran against Ron Clarke." In his talk to us he discussed how on the plane trip over he was pondering the lessons about fitness and aging. He recalled that once, late in his career, he was running with the world record holder Sebastian Coe. They started out even, but finally Coe pulled ahead to win. The lesson Ron took from this was "It is the person who slows down last who wins." This was a perfect life comment. Part of the plan is to set the destination and the course, know how far you have to go, and then *don't slow down.*

Until recently we lacked a sufficient fund of basic information from which planning might proceed with reasonable success. Clearly, planning based on wrong data won't get you very far. Effort must be rewarded with some success, eventually if not initially, or it will extinguish. As someone wise noted, "It's not how many times you fall down that matters, it's how many times you stand up."

The newly found ability to create the future is a direct byproduct of having the necessary smarts to plan. Fate is no longer an acceptable gameplan. Each of us has the moral responsibility to play all four quarters of our life game. At the end of the game we should not be called out on strikes; we should go down swinging. The answer, in simple terms, is that we need resourcefulness and rigor, energy and commitment. Good luck in life becomes a predictable result of laying a good foundation, then sustaining the momentum toward the prophecy that has been set out. Sustaining effort over the course is inherent.

Life is the one game you win by finishing last. Plan for it!

Chapter 6

Ninety-nine Steps to 100

D—DIET

1. Eat to Reach 100
2. Read Well to Eat Well
3. Know When to Eat
4. Know Food and Body Calories
5. Be Fat Alert
6. Count Cholesterol
7. Push Carbos
8. Examine the Pros and Cons of Protein
9. Don't Dry Up
10. A Little Salt Will Do You
11. Keep Your Fiber Up
12. Take Care with Vitamins— Enough Is Enough
13. Calcium Matters
14. Take a Coffee Break
15. Look at Alcohol: Foe and Friend
16. Watch for Chemical Cuisine
17. Beware of Free Radicals
18. Use Your Diet to Fight Cancer

A—ATTITUDE

19. Believe in 100
20. Be Necessary
21. Find Meaning
22. Be an Optimist
23. Take Risks
24. Stay in Control

25. Maintain the Creative Spark
26. Seek Wisdom
27. Be a Responsible Ager
28. Have Options
29. Be a Good Neighbor
30. Cherish Experience
31. Get High on Helping
32. Learn to Learn
33. Don't Kill Yourself
34. Keep Your Senses Sharp
35. Train Your Brain
36. Build Memory
37. Keep Order
38. Be Attractive
39. Recognize That Sex is for Life
40. Stay in Touch
41. Take RX Pet
42. Keep Family Strong
43. Don't Take Yourself so Seriously
44. Work With Stress
45. Have Time Sense
46. Know Your Primary Doctor
47. Pamper Your Glands
48. Be a Good Loser
49. Stay in Tune
50. Stay on the Road
51. Recognize Depression
52. Die Well
53. Have Guts

R — RENEWAL

54. Recharge Yourself
55. Stay in Flow
56. Renew Your Health
57. Cherish Your World
58. Think Travel
59. Think When, Where, and Why Retire
60. Make Your Last Nest Your Best
61. Beware of Retirement Myths
62. Afford Retirement
63. Have a Life Money Plan
64. Be Wealth Fit—Save
65. Keep Working
66. Spend It All
67. Lobby for Yourself
68. Use Leisure
69. Relearn, Rethink, Reeducate
70. Sleep Enough
71. Keep in Rhythm
72. Steps for the Woman
73. Steps for the Man

E — EXERCISE

74. Take the First Step
75. Know How Hard, How Long, How Often to Exercise
76. Realize It's Never Too Late
77. Make Time for Exercise
78. When Tired, Exercise
79. Don't Fear Exercise
80. Don't Say, "I Don't Want to Lose It, But It Hurts Too Much to Use It"
81. Watch Your Fuel Gauge
82. Learn with What and When to Fuel the Exercise
83. Keep Your Oxygen Tanks Full
84. Make Exercise Your Circulation's Best Friend
85. Keep Strong
86. Stay Loose
87. Stay Balanced
88. Stand Straight
89. Work Dem Bones
90. Respect Your Back
91. Honor Your Neck
92. Keep Breathing
93. Use Your Brain—Exercise
94. Chase the Blues
95. Be Sexy, Be Fit
96. Avoid the Big C— Exercise
97. Walk Away from Infection
98. Know that Aging Is Incurable
99. You Don't Have to Win

So you decided you want to live to be 100. After all, it beats the alternative. But it is scarcely a sure bet. Once you've set this goal your chances are immeasurably better if you have a good plan.

This chapter represents my longevity strategy, and the ninety-nine steps I've divided it into represent the difference between usual downhill aging and successful ideal aging.

The steps are grouped not in any priority order, although I would nominate step 19 as the most important. To make 100, you first must believe. Once you believe, the rest follows. But not in any particular order, and not in any particular time. Although it is clearly best to make the effort to dare to be 100

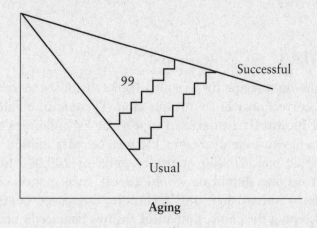

FIG. 9. 99 Steps to Successful Aging.

as early in life as possible, it is never too late to start. The renewal capacity of the human organism is almost boundless.

Because these ninety-nine steps are not a logical sequence, you can start anywhere you want. Some are more important for some people than others, but I'd like to think that each step contains something relevant to everyone. Certainly these steps are not the last word in successful aging, and I hope that if you want more information on any particular topic, you'll turn to the reference sources at the end of the book.

The steps are arranged according to the DARE format, with only loose groupings of steps within each category. If I have left anything out that you think is important, for heaven's sake include it, but don't skip any of these steps. Getting there is all of the fun. The total program is meant to be instructional, but I would hope that you might derive some glimmer of inspiration from it as well. My Dad taught me as a little boy that the wise person deals from the position of strength, and having the smarts to know how makes having the guts to try easier and more logical.

DIET

⌐⌐ **STEP 1.** Eat to Reach 100

What is the right recipe for living to 100? Obviously, there is
no single correct answer to this question. There is an infinite
variety of foodstuffs available to supply the 70 million calories you will consume over your lifetime. Seventy million is
25,000 apple pies, 70,000 quarts of milk, or 200,000 hot
dogs, but no one should or would choose such monotony.
We all eat a varied diet, and the more varied the better,
because keeping the choices plentiful ensures balanced nutrition of high quality.

The other major identifying feature of humans' eating
habits is the dissociation between movement and food. All
other creatures have to move to eat—in fact, their survival is
tightly linked to their ability to find, chase, and digest. Our
survival depends only on imagination and finances.

So what is the right diet to reach 100? It depends on how
much you move. If you are caged (as zoo animals are), then
much restraint is called for. For most beasts of nature, getting
enough to eat is a problem; for us, it is not taking in too much.
Bigger, younger, and more active people are at an advantage.
Because of their higher caloric needs, there is more latitude
with regard to food choices. Conversely, however, small, old,
or inactive people must construct their diets with care. No
matter your size, however, the more you move, the better your
body will utilize your food intake.

A number of obstacles may stand in the way of eating to
reach 100. These obstacles involve dental, exercise, social, and
psychological issues. Poor dentures, financial hardship, isolation, and depression all play substantial roles in the challenge
of eating to be 100. The answer to each deficiency may be
simple and obvious in the abstract, but real-life situations may

occur to overwhelm the simple and obvious answers to these problems. Still, each challenge must be confronted. As an example, ill-fitting dentures may be the insidious culprit that lops a decade of good life off a person's destiny. Such issues need to be confronted intelligently and boldly.

To the rescue comes science. Despite its huge importance in our well-being, our knowledge of nutrition is far from complete. We think we know what a good diet is for a 20-year-old, but is that the same as a 40- or a 60- or a 100-year-old? Ignorance of changing nutritional needs is being replaced by increasingly informed choice. And new food labels should help us eat even better.

So remember, keep food choices varied, and keep moving.

⌐ STEP 2. Read Well to Eat Well

There is every reason to believe that your health is shaped to a major degree by what and how much you put in your mouth.

As you were growing up, you relied on your mother to teach you what you ought to eat. It didn't work. Now the government enters to pick up where Mother let you down. If the Feds fail in their effort to replace motherhood, it isn't for lack of trying.

In 1990 the Nutrition Labeling and Education Act was enacted. Its specific goal was to make food labels more easily understood. Basic information, such as caloric number, calorie type (particularly fat), and content of all additives is mandated. The 400-plus pages of the new regulations attempt to make food choices comprehensible and to diminish the opportunities for "creative" labeling by the manufacturers. For example, the precise amount of actual fruit and vegetable juice in juice drinks must now be labeled.

Numerous terms such as "free," "low," "light," and "fresh" are, by government regulation, specifically defined.

Health claims for food values in regard to specific conditions, such as osteoporosis or high cholesterol levels, are tightly monitored. All of this labeling is indexed to standard portion sizes, not in terms of weight or volume.

The driving principle behind the new food labels is to increase your ability to understand what really goes in your mouth. Of course, labels are not guarantees. It is still up to you to be smart enough to know the few basic steps to healthy nutrition and the incentives to use them.

Clearly you need to get in the habit. As you look at a food selection, you need to pay attention not only to the price, but also to the label: What really is it that you are buying? You need to revise your shopping habits to include another step that evaluates the nutritional value or danger of the components of every meal. Being an informed purchaser and provider is being responsible. And a knowledgeable gourmet is far preferable to an ignorant one.

A secondary benefit of the new labeling regulations should be that the food industry will embark on a program to give you healthier food. A recent survey of food producers indicated that 70 percent are currently doing research on ways to make their products healthier. After all, it is not the outside of the container that is important, it is the inside. Any incentive to help you consumers become more food smart is clearly beneficial. Even Mother would agree to that.

STEP 3. Know When to Eat

When you eat is just as important as what and how you eat. The standard American meal pattern consists of a cup of coffee for breakfast, a sandwich and a soda for lunch, and then a mound of food for dinner. This gorging meal pattern would do a lion proud, but is it right for you?

There is a fund of knowledge that says a gorging meal pattern raises cholesterol levels. Thirty years ago Clarence

Cohn at the University of Chicago fed some volunteers a diet eaten as one meal, others a diet of meals spaced through the day. The results showed that the nibblers had lower cholesterol values. From these findings, Cohn extrapolated that this may be a reason why women, at least early in life, have lower cholesterol levels than men—they tend to be grazers, whereas men tend to be gorgers.

After a meal containing carbohydrates, those potato, fruit, or cereal calories are preferentially used as the body's fuel. But three hours later the body turns to burning its fat as fuel. By eating frequent carbo snacks, you limit this traffic in fat, and thereby protect against higher cholesterol levels.

A more studied reason to have a grazing diet also concerns carbohydrates. If you dump the majority of your calories into your system at one time of day, you impose a heavy instantaneous metabolic burden. Your digestive enzymes and hormones, particularly insulin, have a lot of major work to do in a short time interval. Their response is, with luck, precisely tuned to the challenge, but if there is any oversquirt, say of insulin, then the rise in blood sugar after a big meal is overcompensated for and the result is a rapid drop in blood sugar, called reactive hypoglycemia.

The body is comprised of a whole set of intersecting and complementary functions, which vary over the twenty-four-hour span. You function best when these cycles are mellow, shallow, and frequent, instead of experiencing a single jolt, after which your body spends the remainder of the day trying to catch up.

Of course, the fact that small meals taken throughout the day are better for you than infrequent monster meals does not mean that a Thanksgiving extravagance is harmful. Holidays are holidays. Enjoy. It is the months and years of extra indulgence that are dangerous. So to eat right, learn to be a nibbler.

⌐ **STEP 4.** Know Food and Body Calories

A calorie is a piece of energy. Strictly defined, one calorie is the amount of energy needed to raise the temperature of one liter of water by one degree. A piece of pie at 300 calories, if fully burned by a machine, would raise the temperature of 300 liters of water by 1° C. Of course, you only care about how many calories you need to run your body. Just like any machine, just the right number makes you run the best. However, you should keep in mind that you need calories not just to run your machine, but also to help you grow and repair.

As you age, your calorie needs seem to decrease. Sixteen percent of people over 60 eat fewer than 1,000 calories a day. Is this because they are getting older or because they are less active? Probably both, but mostly because they are less active. As a young person, you may require two or three times as much food and energy as you do at older ages. Clearly, then, if you continue to eat the same amount at older ages as you did when you were young, you will get fat. The fat content of older people's bodies is higher than that of younger people, both because of the calorie excess and because the muscles have deteriorated from decades of underuse.

You should be interested in both the calories in your food and the calories in your body. Having more calories in your body in the form of fat is valuable to your survival only in two extremely rare situations—prolonged starvation and extreme cold. A fat person will outlive a lean one in these situations only.

It takes about a calorie per minute just to keep your basic machinery running, or about 1,500 calories a day. Of course, everyone's needs differ, and your calorie need could go up to 5,000 calories per day if you are very active. This energy must come from food. How well you manage this energy transaction determines how efficient your weight control will be. And remember that you absorb virtually all of the calories you eat.

It is critical to know, too, that a pound of body fat (mine, yours, beef) contains 3,500 calories. This means that in order to gain a pound of fat, you must over some span of time eat 3,500 calories more than your body needs. Conversely, when you seek to lose a pound of fat, you must eat 3,500 calories less than you need to maintain a constant weight.

For example, a 60-year-old woman of moderate activity may require 2,000 calories per day to maintain her weight, but she is ten pounds too heavy and desires a calorie restricted program. To go really slowly on the diet, she takes in 1,800 calories per day, 200 calories a day less than she needs. This means it will take seventeen or eighteen days for her to lose one pound, or six months to lose all ten. But better slow than never.

The new food labels help you to understand better the energy content of what you feed yourself. In 1993, 68 percent of Americans (55 percent of doctors) were overweight. A few of them will make 100, but your chances are much better if your belt is notched in.

STEP 5. Be Fat Alert

Fat is the most energy rich of the three foodstuffs; it yields 9 calories per gram, whereas carbohydrate and protein yield 4 calories per gram. Therefore, a food that contains fat has much more caloric energy content than one with little or no fat. One large Snickers bar has as much fat (200 calories) as 50 apples or 120 potatoes. All foods are fattening, but some more so than others. Because of its richness, it is said that fat makes you fat. It is possible to become fat on carbohydrates, but the basic rule is that it is the fat in your diet that makes your waistline bulge.

Fat is the way your body stores extra calories. A person who is thirty pounds overweight will hold 100,000 extra calories in those fat depots. It sounds like a lot, and it is. For

that reason, it is important to have a long time line in design-
ing corrective dieting. On average, older women's bodies contain about 45 percent body fat. It should be only 25 percent.
Older men's body fat is 35 percent of weight. It should be only
15 percent. It has been calculated that every pound of excess
body weight over ten costs you one month of life.

The American diet currently gets 37 percent of its total
calories from fat, while the recommended proportion should
be 30 percent max. Perhaps even more important is the type of
fats ingested. Fat is classified according to how saturated or
unsaturated it is. These terms refer to the chemical nature of
fat, whether it has a full complement of hydrogen atoms
(saturated) or a relative lack of hydrogen atoms (unsaturated).
Fundamentally, saturated fats are solid, and unsaturated fats
are liquid. Nevertheless, they all contain the same amount of
caloric energy. Ultimately, the critical distinction between the
two is that the effect of saturated fat on raising blood cholesterol levels is more dramatic.

Therefore, although fat is calorically rich, it is the saturated fats that are bad for your cholesterol. Saturated fats are
found predominantly in the animal sources of meat and milk
products. The National Research Council recommends that
no more than 10 percent of daily calories come from animal
fat sources.

Ancel Keys, one of the pioneer nutritionists in the cholesterol field, devised a formula that predicts the effect of a given
dietary fat on cholesterol levels. Most important are the animal saturated fats, which are harmful; next in terms of importance are the unsaturated vegetable oils, which may even help
lower the cholesterol; and least important is the actual cholesterol in our diets, which, again, raises the blood levels. The
NRC recommends no more than 300 mg total cholesterol per
day, usually found in egg yolks. The wise intake for eggs seems
to be no more than four per week.

The Prudent Diet says: Reduce the diet fat load.

Choose lean meats. Use more poultry, fish.
Remove visible fat (e.g., skin from chicken).
Broil/bake; don't fry.
Replace meat with vegetables.
Use low-fat/no-fat milk and cheese.
Watch the dressing, dips, popcorn butter.

Increase exercise, avoid fat triggers, reward yourself (but not with fatty foods) for pounds lost and cholesterol levels lowered.

STEP 6. Count Cholesterol

Cholesterol is not all bad. In fact, you'd be in a bad way without it, as it is a vital part of all your cells. It's just that you have too much. The simplest way to measure it is through your blood, since it gives a rough approximation of the amount in your arteries, which is where the problem lies. The accepted normal range is below 200 mg per 100 cc of blood. Where did this watermark come from? It is clearly a statistical figure, since the blood cholesterol value of the Kalahari Bushmen (whose current lifestyle is similar to that of 2 million years ago) is 77 mg per 100 cc. Not surprisingly, there is no hardening of the arteries noted in these people. Contemporary cholesterol values are therefore roughly three times higher than that in the past—no wonder we're clogged up with it.

The cholesterol in your body comes and goes, which is why the amount in your arteries can be gotten rid of through a rigid program of lowering. Seventy percent of your cholesterol comes from that which you yourself manufacture, mostly in the liver; only one third comes directly from the diet. This is why a low-cholesterol diet is not as important as a cholesterol-lowering diet.

As it exists in your body, most cholesterol serves as a way to dissolve fat; in essence it helps absorb and transport fat. So the more fat your liver sees, either in the diet or from the fat in your body (as with stress), the more cholesterol it makes. This phenomenon explains why accountants' cholesterol values go up early in April, and med students' levels go up at exam time.

The cholesterol story becomes more complex with the discovery that not all cholesterol is bad for you. The high-density lipoprotein (HDL) cholesterol actually seems good for you. The famous Framingham Heart Health Study has clearly shown that those of us with high HDL levels seem protected against heart disease, and those with low levels are at really high risk, despite what the total cholesterol level is. For example, I would rather have a patient with a total cholesterol of 240 with an HDL of 60 than a patient with a cholesterol of 200 with an HDL of 30. The major factors that seem to increase the HDL cholesterol levels are physical exercise and a moderate intake of alcohol. So, strange as it might sound, the drinking jogger seems to be favored.

There has been much discussion, too, whether it is still advisable to try to lower the cholesterol levels in people over 65. Several strong studies suggest that it is. I welcome this perspective, as I have held to the idea that age alone should not be the criterion for development of passive attitudes about health promotion. This does not mean that older persons, particularly those 75 or older, who are always at risk for restriction of dietary diversity, should be further confined by a rigid diet aimed at getting the blood cholesterol down. But I stand firm in my conviction that it is never too late to be as healthy as possible, and this means having as low cholesterol and as high an HDL level as is possible, no matter your age.

STEP 7. Push Carbos

Carbohydrates are pure energy. Unlike fat and protein, which serve as part of your structure, the job of carbohydrates is almost exclusively to fuel your metabolism. After a meal, nearly all your energy comes from carbohydrates. When you don't eat for a while, the body turns to its fat stores to run the machinery, but over a whole day it's the carbos that keep you going.

The body has a relatively small storage tank of carbohydrates—only a few thousand calories at most—so you need to keep restocking it from the foods you eat. The newly formulated food pyramid, advanced by the National Research Council, advocates that you eat five servings of fruit and vegetables per day, and six to eleven servings of cereal and grain products. This then leads to a diet in which approximately 55 percent of calories will come from carbohydrates.

Dietary carbohydrates come in three sizes: simple, compound, and complex. The simple carbohydrates include table sugar, a small molecule with six carbon atoms and a bunch of hydrogen and oxygen for company. Compound carbos are the fruit sugars, in which two simple sugars are chemically bonded to contain twelve carbon atoms plus hydrogen and oxygen. Complex carbos contain maybe hundreds of simple sugars clumped together like a latticework. These are the starches of vegetables and grains.

It is important to recognize that for your body to burn a potato for energy, the complex carbohydrates must be totally broken down to the simple sugars of which it is basically made. In a sense, therefore, a potato or piece of bread ultimately becomes sugar before it is used. But before this bread or potato is burned, it takes a while for the body to break down the complex structure of its molecules; conversely, simple sugars can enter your cells in a rush and flood the cells' machinery with a sugar push.

The most common defect in the body's ability to use carbohydrates is diabetes, which has two forms. The first, which is less common and is termed juvenile diabetes, results from the destruction of the pancreas's ability to make insulin, which facilitates sugar's usage. The more common form, adult onset diabetes, develops, in my view, as a result of lack of exercise and consequent fat gain, leading to the relative inability to use blood sugar for energy. The answer to the first form is insulin, whereas the answer to the second is exercise and weight loss.

A high-carbohydrate diet has the advantage of great diversity and low cost. Fruits, vegetables, and grains also carry with their energy provision high levels of important micronutrients, vitamins, and minerals. The simple sugars, however, are known to be "empty calories." That is, they provide "only" pure energy without the other good stuff. Your diet derives 20 percent of its calories from simple sugar. Your sweet tooth is an evolutionary residue from your aboriginal days, when the only natural sweet was honey, again a concentrated energy source and therefore prized. Now sugar is all too readily available as a part of your food offering.

The 3 million vegetarians in this country tend to live a long time. This has to mean something. Also, the fact that champion athletes carbo load before an important athletic event must mean that an increased carbohydrate presence should be in your kitchen and dining room.

STEP 8. Examine the Pros and Cons of Protein

Protein is who you are. Your brain, your heart, your muscles are mostly protein. It is your flesh and blood, 60 percent of your dry weight.

Protein in turn consists of amino acids, relatively simple compounds made up of carbon, hydrogen, oxygen, nitrogen, and some sulfur. Only twenty-two of these basic amino acids constitute, in innumerable combinations, all the millions of types of protein in the world.

There are eight of the amino acids that your body cannot make and therefore must be part of your diet—the "essential" amino acids. The most secure way to obtain these essential amino acids is by eating a meat diet. This is not to say that meat is the only source of the essential eight, as they are also present in some plant foods, particularly legumes. A vegetarian who is wise and well instructed can totally fulfill the basic amino acid need with a well-conceived collection of vegetables.

There has developed a substantial backlash against the meat-and-potato diet of a few decades ago, partly driven by health concerns, the rest by environmental issues. The health concerns derive largely from the fact that most meat is highly prized, not just for its protein content, but because it also contains fat. The marbling of prime meats costs more, both in cash and health. Many studies show that those rich countries which have a high meat (fat) intake have a high incidence of heart disease.

As you age, you need to keep your protein intake high to help offset the loss of muscle tissue. This is often a problem because meat tends to be more expensive and harder to prepare and digest, particularly by people with dental problems. Age, too, is accompanied by disease states that impose their own added requirements for protein. Therefore, as we age, protein, particularly as lean meats, low-fat milk, and legumes, should be maintained at relatively high levels.

PROTEIN RATINGS OF COMMON FOODS	
Eggs	100
Fish	70
Lean beef	70
Milk	60
Rice	57
Soybeans	50
Potatoes	35

One of the most important blood tests as you grow older is that which tracks the albumin level in the blood. Albumin is the most important protein in the blood, and its level is sensitive to the adequacy of protein nutrition. If albumin levels become too low, extra foods high in protein content are recommended.

During the traditional American holidays, meat dishes are often the centerpiece of family banquets, and this festive component of eating should not be neglected—particularly when it also happens to be good for you.

_ſ_ STEP 9. Don't Dry Up

Almost none of us pay much attention to the amount of fluid we drink—it's just a part of our lives that takes care of itself. Right? Wrong. The recommended daily allowance for water proposed by the National Research Council is a quart and a half a day. Few of us have ever intentionally drunk a quart and a half just because we are supposed to. Our wonderful kidneys let us get away with such nonchalance as they carefully regulate the amount of fluid we excrete or retain according to how much we drink. The kidneys filter 150 quarts of blood per day, but excrete only 1 percent of this. The urine our kidneys makes serves as a transfer vehicle for some of the waste materials of our bodies, particularly the urea derived from protein metabolism.

But when we get older, our cuing becomes faulted. In other words, when older people are denied fluid for twenty-four hours, their thirst response is blunted. We sometimes drink when we shouldn't, causing dilution of our body minerals, or we don't drink when we should, which causes dehydration. Medicines—particularly diuretics—and disease conditions often seen in older people make fluid consumption more than a casual affair. Neglect of symptoms and poor compliance with medications can be very dangerous. Severe constipation can also complicate dehydration.

Our hunter-gatherer ancestors only had water to drink.

Nowadays, however, it seems almost no able-bodied person drinks plain water. Fluid comes in various colors and temperatures, with varying bubbles and other companions. But water still claims many advantages. It has no calories, it has no salt, and it does its job of lubricating us just fine. We are, after all, 60 percent water.

Then there are the external factors. Heat causes increased fluid loss through perspiration, which can, on occasion, be extreme and result in substantial dehydration. Infection, when accompanied by fever, clearly imposes an increased fluid demand, and colds in particular benefit from more fluid intake, as fluids help keep the mucus from getting too sticky and difficult to eliminate. The aging process itself has been shown to disrupt the body's thermoregulatory center, so fluid ingestion when the temperature rises is very important. That's why heat waves are dangerous for older people.

Of course, fluids are not the only source of body water, as your food produces almost as much and your metabolism generates a smaller amount. So, if you don't eat well for any one of a number of reasons, dehydration may result. Your body can stand weeks of calorie loss, but your fluid reserves are at more immediate risk.

Another complication seen in older persons that can cause fluid distress is the annoying need to urinate at night, causing disruption in sleep. Many older persons respond by simply not drinking enough. This misadventure is best addressed by making sure you drink enough fluid early in the day, so that the bladder doesn't have to perform so much at night. Drink early, drink enough, and never let your urine turn dark due to dehydration.

STEP 10. A Little Salt Will Do You

You are not a freshwater creature. You are a saltwater creature. All your cells live in a salty lake, like the oceans where life first evolved. The salt content of your body fluids is two teaspoonfuls per quart.

With civilization has come the increased availability of salt at cheap prices. We have learned to use salt at almost every step of the food process, from preservation to processing, preparation, and consumption.

Your salt intake varies from one to fifteen teaspoonfuls per day. This is in contrast to what your hunter-gatherer ancestors ate, around a quarter teaspoonful. Ordinarily, your kidneys manage to balance the varied amount of salt you take against the need for that day. During a bout of diarrhea, which depletes you rapidly of a lot of salt, or on a very heavy sweating day, during which two teaspoonfuls can be lost in the sweat, your kidneys shut down salt excretion to prevent further loss. Conversely, when you consume a heavier than average load, the kidneys simply get rid of it.

But what if the balancing act is imperfect? What if too much is lost or too much is saved? If the concentration of sodium in your body fluids becomes too low as the result of excess sweating, or vomiting, or diarrhea, you become weak, confused, and even delirious. If your sodium content is too acutely high, you become dehydrated. If it is chronically high, you can develop high blood pressure.

There is clear evidence that in those countries in which salt intake is high, particularly Japan, incidence of high blood pressure is exaggerated. A further compounding feature is obesity, a condition in which the kidneys seem particularly prone to hold onto salt. Therefore, being overweight and eating a lot of salt in your diet is a bad idea. The picture becomes even worse if you're underexercising, because exercise in and of itself protects against high blood pressure. The worst combination, then, is the underexercised fat person who eats a lot of salt.

To prevent this predicament, stay slim, exercise, and watch your salt intake. A minimal requirement per day is about a quarter teaspoonful. Never salt before tasting. Use pepper, garlic or onion powder, or herbs as substitutes. Don't put the salt shaker on the table. Beware of convenience foods, as they are usually thick with salt. Also be aware that many medicines, particularly those given for the treatment of arthritis, have a marked tendency to promote the body's salt retention. Read food labels. Eat fresh foods that have very little salt. And use only half of the salt called for in recipes.

⌐ STEP 11. Keep Your Fiber Up

Fiber is the skeleton of plants and fruits. It gives them their architecture. Plants are made up mostly of fiber.

The Western diet—with its emphasis on processed animal foods—is fiber poor. The typical American diet may contain 12 grams per day, whereas diets in Third World countries may contain ten times as much. For millions of years our ancestors ate only uncooked food, largely roots and shoots. They had healthy intestines.

Fiber has no calories, and it is not absorbed by your gut. It comes in two varieties, the soluble and insoluble, both of which have positive health benefits. First, fiber decreases the incidence of different types of cancer by speeding the transit time of food in your intestine and diluting potential carcinogens. Second, it cuts down diverticulosis (the little pockets commonly found bulging off the colon in older people) and hemorrhoids. Third, it helps prevent constipation. I recall a fancy scientific lecture I attended in Boston a few years ago on the intestinal problems of older people. The speaker went on for the better part of an hour, but the punch line at the end concerned the secret for good bowel habit: "prunes." Fourth, it helps control weight by its bulk and ability to satiate, substituting for high-calorie foods. Finally, and maybe most important, fiber is a major aid in lowering blood cholesterol. The soluble kind of fiber acts like a blotter in the intestines, helping absorb fat and cholesterol, and facilitating their excretion. This welcome effect of soluble fiber on cholesterol levels is also separate and above that of decreasing dietary fat. Said in another way, if you can lower your cholesterol 20 points by cutting fat, including soluble fiber will decrease it by another 20 points.

Fiber can be fun. The *Tufts Diet and Nutrition Letter* of March 1994 lists a whole bunch of interesting fiber options, including barley, couscous, and millet, that can add interest and variety to your foods.

Although regular foods are the preferred way of guaranteeing more dietary fiber, there are also a number of proprietary preparations available that all contain psyllium, a purified seed fiber product. These work in the same way as natural fiber, and they are frequently recommended by gastroenterologists for their older patients who may be confronted with any of the conditions noted above.

As you age, you should keep the fiber content of your diets high. The advantages are many, and the practice is cheap and safe.

⌐ STEP 12. Take Care with Vitamins— Enough Is Enough

Vitamins are like light switches. You need a certain number to light your house. Following the same analogy, having ten or a hundred times that number doesn't make the lights any brighter. Vitamins, unlike food substances, are not, in effect, used up. They act as catalysts to help metabolism happen, but they are regenerated in the process. Consequently, they are needed only in minimal amounts—just like light switches.

You need thirteen different vitamin catalysts. Four of them are fat soluble (A, D, E, and K), and the other nine are water soluble. The fat-soluble ones are stored in your tissues, and all the others (including all the B vitamins) must be supplied on a regular basis, as they are not stored.

Seventy million Americans feel they need more light switches in their lives, but most don't. Vitamin fever is fed by diets of fast burgers, fries, and sodas, all of which have little vitamin value. As an antidote to the quick eat, many resort to vitamins to offset the guilt of other dereliction. The best guilt salve, however, is fruits and vegetables. If everyone ate fruits and vegetables instead of junk plus vitamins, the vitamin craze would have little to justify it.

The central truth of good nutrition is that your needs are best met by a varied and complex diet. As you age, however, your total calorie need often falls, so what was an easily balanced diet, say, on a 2,500-calorie daily intake becomes a problem when the calorie count drops to 1,500. I often prescribe vitamins to older patients, particularly if I feel they are at risk for not eating the traditional well-balanced menu. Perhaps one quarter of older people get by with fewer than 1,000 calories a day.

When I do suggest vitamins, I encourage comparison shopping to be sure that these inexpensive compounds are not "glitzed up." A balanced multivitamin tablet or capsule should cost only a few cents. Also, I discourage the ultra high-potency formulas as unnecessary and almost always too expensive. Vitamins also lose shelf potency, so buy them fresh. Furthermore, megadoses of vitamins can be dangerous. There is no evidence that consumption of megavitamins improves exercise performance or has any beneficial effects on the aging process.

Common sense and economics dictate that nutritional salvation is unlikely to emerge from any pill bottle. Vitamin pills are the last resort, leaving good food the first choice. I have never yet met or tasted a vitamin as satisfying to eye or palate as a fruit, vegetable, meat, or grain.

⌐⌐ **STEP 13.** Calcium Matters

Of all the body's minerals, calcium is the most important. We would all be jellyfish without it. It not only gives your bones their sturdiness (as steel does for buildings), but it also serves as a vital participant in innumerable bodily chemical reactions. It helps muscles contract, the heart to beat, and the brain to think. All in all, your body contains about three and a half pounds of calcium.

Clearly, you need the right amount of calcium in your diet and your body. Generally, if you need more calcium your gut traps more, and your kidneys excrete less. But this protective system has many flaws. The calcium in your bones declines at a rate of about 1 to 3 percent per year.

Counterstrategies may modify this. For instance, countries whose inhabitants consume more dairy products also have citizens with more calcium in their bones. But diet is only a part of the story. There is almost no osteoporosis in Third World countries—not necessarily because of high dairy product intake, but because of the high levels of physical exercise. Fractured hips are a disease of inactivity and diminished calcium intake. Twenty-five million Americans have osteoporosis. Women are particularly at risk, having three to five times as many problems from weak bones as men.

The recommended dietary allowance for calcium is 1,500 milligrams per day, the equivalent of three glasses of milk. Even early in life, however, most of us don't reach this ideal, so bone loss starts frequently in the 20s, but does not become pronounced enough to result in fractures until the 70s and beyond. Milk and its derivatives are the principal source of dietary calcium, but fish, particularly sardines, and green vegetables (broccoli, spinach) supply it as well.

Unfortunately, calcium intake tends to decrease as you grow older. Whether this is a matter of taste or the avoidance of milk products due to a condition known as lactose intolerance (which results in diarrhea after consumption of a dairy product) is unknown. In any case, calcium supplementation through any number of food or over-the-counter products is highly advised.

I have treated hundreds of older people, mostly women, with fractured hips. Fractured hips are major nuisances in and of themselves, but more importantly may result in further decreased physical activity and independence, leading to a downward spiral in life quality. In thinking about how such situations could have been prevented, one truism stands out. Active people don't break easily. Most hip fractures I encounter are not the result of a big fall, but rather that of an awkward step off a curb or slip off the sofa. Such casual insults end up in 250,000 fractured hips and 500,000 fractured vertebrae every year. And to add more insult to injury, the rest required after a fracture increases calcium loss by fiftyfold. Why risk it?

It is never too late to take calcium and start exercising, and prevent fractures that can hamper your lifestyle.

STEP 14. Take a Coffee Break

One million tons of coffee are consumed each year in the United States. That's ten pounds for each person, an average of four cups per day. We are a nation high on coffee beans. The coffee break, a cultural obsession, comes in all sorts of new boutique forms.

The active ingredient of coffee, caffeine, serves to get your juices going. It is the predominant central nervous system stimulant, often obscuring, for a while at least, your chronically sleep-deprived state. A cup of coffee may contain 50 to 150 mg of caffeine, a cup of tea 10 to 50 mg, and a cola soft drink 50 mg. Caffeine has been shown to improve athletic performance, and is classified as a "controlled substance" by the Olympic Organizing Committee.

But this rush comes at some cost. I can feel my blood sugar surging and plunging in phase with a previous cup of coffee. I like the high but hate the low. For this reason, coffee use by diabetics must be carefully monitored. Coffee is also tough on people who carry a lot of stress in their lives, because the jangle of life and its natural challenges can be made more acute by a caffeine load. Many long and restless nights can be attributed to coffee consumption. Ulcers in the intestine are aggravated by coffee ingestion, as gastric acid goes up after coffee consumption. Not surprisingly, many bellyaches have been helped merely by the restriction of coffee intake.

Coffee also acts as a diuretic. Not only does coffee provide a fluid load, but caffeine acts to increase blood flow to the kidneys, thereby increasing fluid loss even more. As you age, this feature is of substantial importance, as you try to minimize fluctuations in your fluid balance.

It is the cardiovascular system that has been most studied with regard to coffee drinking. There is no question that for the casual (not the hard-core) coffee buff, the pulse rate goes up and the blood pressure rises. As consumption—and tolerance—builds up, these effects are blunted. Ten years or so ago, a number of scientific reports seemed to indicate that coffee drinking increases serum cholesterol levels and causes heart trouble, and so was considered to be a risk factor for coronary disease. These studies have not been confirmed, however.

The consensus today seems to be that coffee, *consumed in moderation,* is not harmful, and its incorporation into your daily life is benign. It's what you put *in* your coffee that can be bad for you.

_⌐ **STEP 15.** Look at Alcohol: Foe and Friend

Sixty-some percent of adult Americans drink alcohol, from which they derive 7 to 10 percent of their calories. Generally speaking, a glass of beer or a mixed drink contains 100 calories. Any effort to control weight must include clear recognition of these calories. True, there is no fat or cholesterol in these calories, but there is almost nothing else of nutritive value either; hence the applicable term, "empty calories."

All of you are aware of the dangers of too much alcohol. Physical damage to the liver, heart, and brain accompany prolonged heavy use. Accident rates are clearly alcohol driven. But the major danger in drinking alcohol is the social disaffection and strained relationships that often accompany it. Several self-directed questions reflect whether alcohol use is getting in your way of reaching 100.

1. Do you use alcohol as a way to settle your nerves?

2. Does your behavior change and make you more angry or depressed when you drink?

3. Do you drink at the same time each day?

4. Are you truthful with yourself about your alcohol use?

5. Are you irresponsible after you drink?

Alcoholism has genetic and behavioral roots. The alcoholic usually has low self-esteem, and his self-control mechanisms are lost. Risk of alcohol abuse increases as you age, because tolerance decreases and disease states and multiple drug interactions pose even further dangers.

Another side to the alcohol story concerns the consecutive reports of benefits of *moderate* alcohol use. The Harvard Health Professional Study of 51,000 persons over an eight-year period has shown a 20 percent decrease in coronary heart disease in those who took one to two drinks per day, and a 40 percent decrease in those who took three to four per day. In 1993 a *New England Journal of Medicine* article similarly reported that three drinks per day seemed to provide a 50 percent protection against heart attacks. A nurses' study seemed to show similar results as those in men.

Our attention was grabbed by the *60 Minutes* report, "The French Paradox," which reported that the French, despite a fat-rich diet, had very low levels of heart disease. This was credited to a heavy consumption of red wine. Whether the benefit is bestowed by a product of grape skin, the alcohol, or something else (such as a different lifestyle) is still open to question. Clearly, however, alcohol has a beneficial effect on good HDL cholesterol levels, and on the clottability of blood.

Yet these stated benefits cannot stand alone. Alcohol can kill as well as aid. The oracle at Delphi seems to have had it right. Everything in moderation. A little is good, too much is a poison.

STEP 16. Watch for Chemical Cuisine

For centuries, people have been messing around with your food. They have tried to preserve it, sterilize it, make it tastier, give it a different color. The widespread use of food additives makes us wonder how we survived before them. Some food is said to be even better for you because of enrichment with vitamins, minerals, or fiber. One commonly heard suggestion is to shop in the outer rims of the supermarket, to guard against the inner aisles—where the processed foods containing most artificial ingredients are displayed. The increased incorporation of additives and processed foods into the diet has led some to near hysteria about their use. As a result, "natural foods" are a growth industry.

Are additives safe? The answer, for the most part, is yes. However, without question a substantial number of people are simply allergic to one or more of the added chemicals. Asthma, hives, and other allergic symptoms may follow a meal laced with food colorings or preservatives or taste enhancers. Most notable of these compounds is monosodium glutamate, or MSG, which is the cause of the so-called Chinese restaurant syndrome (due to the high use of MSG in Chinese dishes). Fortunately, these excess reactions, such as headaches and facial burning, are relatively rare. Other additives are suspected to increase the oxidants—or the carcinogen, hormone, or antibiotic content—in food. What mischief lurks in all of these compounds produced by the chemistry labs of the food industry, whose number one priority is profit?

When you calculate the tons and tons of additives that go into our nation's bellies, it is extraordinary that so few problems seem to have arisen. The most commonly used additives are the sweeteners produced and consumed, seemingly by the tankerload. The diet drink industry is dependent on aspartame (NutraSweet and Equal) and saccharine, two compounds that are two to four hundred times sweeter than sugar. The diets of millions of diabetics have been broadened because of the availability of these substances, which are safe. It is true that a study showed that bladder cancer occurred in rats when they were fed the equivalent of 850 cans of soft drinks per day, but overall the safety record seems very high.

Caffeine is a common additive as well, often added to soft drinks. Not generally recognized, however, is the fact that non-cola drinks may also have added caffeine. Caffeine is mildly addictive and may lead to upper sensations of restlessness, rapid heart beat, and insomnia. Both pregnant women and those with bumpy hearts should avoid caffeinated products.

The most dangerous food additive is bacteria that inadvertently contaminates food during storage or preparation. Several watchwords exist about these organisms:

> Don't buy foods in damaged wrappers.
> Eat hot foods hot.
> Eat cold foods cold.
> Eat all foods in as fresh a form as possible.

Don't overbuy.
Watch for expiration dates.

It is inevitable that your food will continue to go through various steps between its original source and the form it's in when it reaches your stomach. Be vigilant about which steps those are.

⌐ STEP 17. Beware of Free Radicals

One of the major theories of aging, discussed earlier, concerns the production by the body of tiny chemicals called free radicals. A free radical is an unstable and toxic result of your metabolism, inevitable byproducts of your living in an oxygen-risk environment, otherwise known as "molecular terrorists." These pieces of metabolic ash are produced by the hundreds of millions every day in all your body cells.

But your body is too smart to allow this debris to pile up in your cells and has derived a whole set of machinery, the purpose of which is to get rid of this unwelcome stash of oxidized free radicals. Unfortunately, your capacity to rid yourself of these elements goes down as you grow older. The proposition immediately emerges: Why not juice up the protective machinery by taking in compounds known to act as counterterrorists, i.e. the antioxidants?

Antioxidants are a hot item. They are widely featured in health food stores. They are big business. Why *not* bump up your protection by taking extra? A host of studies involved the intake of antioxidants—extra vitamin E, vitamin C, selenium, and so on—to prove that life is extended, or baldness retarded, or potency extended, and so on. Such efforts have drawn a multitude of the faithful to their support, including a large number of health professionals who are eager advocates for the use of antioxidants as health aides.

For every study that shows benefits, however, there is

another study that doesn't. In April 1994 the *New England Journal of Medicine* published a large report on a research project in Finland, in which the antioxidant beta carotene was administered to a group of smokers. Not only did the hopeful compounds not have a beneficial effect, they seemed possibly to be harmful. Those who took beta carotene had 18 percent more lung cancer than those who didn't. So clearly the final verdict isn't in.

The one piece of evidence that influences my perspective the most so far is that numerous efforts to extend the lifespan of experimental animals by the use of free radical scavengers haven't worked. The hypothesis of a vitamin E fountain of youth hasn't held up. I confess an innate resistance to the whole notion that something that comes out of a plastic container can undo the damage caused largely by decades of dereliction of stress and disuse, overconsumption, under-exercise, and general neglect. The easy fix or quick cure goes along with the American psyche, but my gut feeling is that the drugstore is not going to be where you'll shop for health. You are your own best apothecary.

_⌐_ STEP 18. Use Your Diet to Fight Cancer

Most cancer is caused by lightning. It strikes out of the blue. But cancer doesn't just happen by chance. It has a cause. Diet is one of the environmental hazards that lead to cancer—and the evidence for this is manyfold. Some factors in diet seem to cause cancer; others seem to protect against it. You need to be aware of what you put in your stomach if you seek to decrease your chance of encountering malignancy.

For example, the Japanese have twelve times the incidence of stomach cancer as Caucasians, a differential that is strongly held to be due to as yet unidentified dietary factors.

Fat in the diet has been repeatedly linked with breast cancer. Whether it is the fat itself or the calories inherent in high-fat diets is not clear, but when women or men are over-weight, their sex hormone levels are altered in such ways as to bathe the sensitive tissues in higher than average hormone levels. As support of the link between the two, the fact exists that breast cancer is much less common in Third World countries than in the U.S. A study of 48,000 men showed that those who had high dietary fat intake had two and a half times higher incidence of prostate cancer than those with low fat consumption. Colon cancer also shows a correlation between incidence rates and dietary fat consumption. Colon cancer is rare in Africa, but is common in African-Americans; cancer rates for Japanese are similar when they adapt to our diet. Further, a high alcohol consumption appears to encourage esophageal and stomach cancers.

On the other hand, a wide variety of foodstuffs appears to act as a protector against cancer. This range includes fiber, vitamins, and some sulfides contained in garlic and onions. The mode of action of these ingestibles is either supposedly direct or induced by somehow stimulating cancer-fighting enzymes.

Vegetables, greens, and fruits, which are beneficial for other reasons, seem to supply substances that act as cancer shields. Conversely, the fatty foods of meat and milk products are suspected villains.

Despite the studies, however, all the research that indicates an effect of diet on the rate of cancer is indirect. It is based on experiments in test tubes and in animals, and on epidemiological associations. No one has proposed that a certain foodstuff is a direct cure for or protection against malignancy. If such were the case, we would all be taking it or avoiding it. When this major food is discovered, I hope that it is something I like. In the meantime, what makes sense to me is to eat a well-balanced diet with major emphasis on the plant foods. Cancer is cruel. You need to employ constantly emerging information as to diet threats and benefits to limit its assault on you and your family.

ATTITUDE

⌐ **STEP 19.** Believe in 100

The most important step is the first. A journey of a hundred miles or years begins not with the first movement forward, but with the thought that precedes it. "The belief in 100" is so important because you are moldable, shapable like clay under a sculptor's hands—yours. The ultimate challenge of anyone's life is the opportunity to make the most of it that can be made. "To thine own self be true" becomes "to thine own best self be true." Who you get to be—how old, wise, competent, active, creative, sexy, fun you become—depends on how you plan. Decrepitude and loss are not predetermined. How you, like the turtle, set your course is highly predictive of the journey you will take.

How lucky we are to be alive at this time of history! Until now we have had no dependable road maps. We didn't know how far our journey might be, how we should provision ourselves, how many resources we might need, how much gas would carry us the whole way, and what degree of maintenance our vehicle would need to ensure our safe arrival at our final destination.

It is true that an occasional discovery will occur by chance, but far more likely is the situation in which we know where we would like to go, and plan accordingly. Before now, reaching 100 years of age was a mythical prospect. As a young boy, I recall thinking anyone over 70 extremely old. But now 100 years is common. Every month I see someone over 100 in my medical office. Take Clara Willman, age 101. She came in by herself. She still lives by herself and takes full charge of her affairs. She came to my office simply for my approval of her anticipated six-week trip to Minneapolis to be with her family. She would travel alone. I found her as fit and eager as on previous visits and wished her a good trip. When Clara was a little girl, she didn't believe in reaching 100 because she didn't conceive that the possibility existed. She got to this "miraculous" age by accident.

For the rest of us, the fact that she has made it makes it easier for us. The trail is broken and the way shown. As more of us do it, the easier it will be for the rest of us to believe.

One hundred years is not freakish. It is a natural endowment. It can and should be ours, if we don't mess it up, or unless the lightning strikes.

In the *Will to Believe* William James wrote, "Be not afraid of life. Believe that life is worth living, and your belief will help create the fact. It is only by risking your person from one hour to another that you live at all. Your faith beforehand in an uncertified result will make the result come true."

Believe in 100.

STEP 20. Be Necessary

When I was 8 or 9 years old, my Grandpa Bortz said to me, "Make yourself necessary." I have no recall of what prompted this advice nor why I happen to remember it, but fifty-five years later, this small counsel from him has emerged as life shaping.

Dear friend George Sheehan was less modest. His advice was "Make yourself indispensable." George and Grandpa bid each of us to reach deep inside ourselves to find some element that someone or something else needs. Ben E. King sang, "Lean on me." We all need someone to lean on us.

By being necessary, indispensable, useful, each morning means something. This prospect is not at all automatic. My scary guess is that a large number of us gets up in the morning and goes to bed at night without being necessary at all. If this is the case, why live?

Being necessary does not imply an elite role in life. Being older—with the added gifts of experience to offer—makes it easier to be necessary. The examples of people becoming and being necessary into late life are many. Most are quiet little stories that tell of individuals adopting an orphan overseas, leading a singalong at a nursing home, mentoring a troubled kid, volunteering in a hospice unit, being a penpal to someone less fortunate—the opportunities are endless. Being necessary can be as simple as having a pet or doing volunteer work or writing a letter to the editor or picking up litter or enriching the life of your great-great-grandchild by reading to him or her or teaching someone how to knit or helping with the dishes or campaigning for your favorite candidate. When we stop mattering in this world, our continued consumption of resources becomes senseless. And I'm not talking about making money—but simply having a fruitful role in the world to play, being sure you show up when your cue is given.

Being necessary has clear survival advantages. Medical journals are full of evidence that show when a spouse or close partner dies, the endurability of the remaining partner is jeopardized. Married people live longer because marriage implies interdependent relationships. Each is necessary for the other. When this contract is broken and necessity seems at risk, then death lurks.

Being necessary, indispensable, or useful means keeping the energy level up. You can't disengage and be necessary at the same time. You must take risks and remain resourceful. Being necessary means being in sync with the times, being relevant. You can't aspire to be necessary if what you have to offer has no value. Being necessary implies continued growth and synchronicity with the world around you.

⎍ **STEP 21.** Find Meaning

The most important advantage of growing old is the opportunity to search for meaning. A child—or even a 40-year-old—simply hasn't lived long enough, seen enough, hurt and triumphed enough, to develop a sense of the whole. This is the reason old people have been valued so highly in primitive cultures; they have lived long enough to achieve the perspective only time can provide. Their experience was an invaluable survival asset to their tribe.

Until relatively recently, many invoked a supernatural basis for meaning, a belief in a divine design in which we were passive participants. The comfort of this position is less widely shared today. Today a growing number of people are seeking a unifying vision or explanation of how this big universe works, without resorting to metaphysical concepts.

The conventional scientific stance is that life has no intrinsic meaning, that there is no purposeful design in the universe. The stars, planets, canyons, and tadpoles of the universe are because they are, without intentional design or externally driven purpose. This assertion does not imply, however, that our world has no meaning. It simply has no meaning by itself. It must be given meaning by an active and conscious effort to provide it. I propose that purpose and understanding are involved in meaning. For anything or anyone to be thought of as having a meaning, that it or person must demonstrate purpose. Similarly, understanding what the purpose is provides meaning.

It is clear that the present consumption mentality does not bring meaning. Possessions are almost irrelevant to the development of meaning; they may actually get in its way. Early in life, our preoccupation is with self and the narcissistic accumulation of material goods. But as we progress through life, goods become less important. A common observation I find in my old, old patients is their casual indifference to their checking account balance or their acreage.

It is the last life stage that gives you the wonderful opportunity to search for meaning, to take the voyage to yourself, that will lend comprehension to where you have been and the relationship of your time to the cosmic order. Not all old people will reach—or even desire to reach—this platform for survey of the grand panorama of life. With more knowledge and involvement, opportunity for deep understanding appears.

My hope, when I hit 100, is that I will see and understand with clarity what was previously obscured by the inexperience and distortion of early life. This will signify final success.

STEP 22. Be an Optimist

Norman Cousins wrote, "No one is smart enough to be a pessimist." But it is safer and more fashionable. If you waken and say the world is rotten, then you'll never be disappointed, because the world has enough dark recesses to justify this assertion. However, painting the day in dark colors before the sun has a chance to come up prejudges the daylight and makes vivid experience more difficult.

Pessimists set their compass in such a direction as to guarantee the entropic, deteriorative quality of tomorrow's world. Optimists have the chance to do the reverse—to challenge entropy, and through an active force of will, assert the possibility of a more orderly and congenial world. I am constantly fascinated by the emerging reports from the neurology laboratories of the world that reveal how the brain responds to different environmental signals, changing its structure to make it more responsive to those signals. Since this is the way your most important organ seems to work, it makes sense to me that you train your brain to be positive. You practice seeing the bright side. You eliminate the negative. You create circuitry within your brain to position each morning to reveal opportunity instead of threat. As Albert Einstein observed, "An optimist has green lights all day long. The pessimist has red."

Optimism can be learned. Of course, the optimist must beware that merely setting a course along the compass point in no way guarantees the arrival at the desired destination. But not to set the course at all gives little if any chance of success. Optimism appears as a moral imperative.

It is my optimistic forecast that knowledge is the key to optimism. Two trite truisms are "Ignorance is bliss" and "What you don't know can't hurt you." Both are miserably wrong. Ignorance creates entirely the wrong atmosphere for having a good day. It is knowledge and the confidence it inspires that allows the dawn to arrive full of hope. We are afraid of what we don't know. The more we know— particularly about the almost limitless potentials of being human—the more we are empowered and the brighter the world is. We know more confidently what we can and can't do, and also the difference between the two.

When we become smart, we become optimists. It is an imperative.

STEP 23. Take Risks

The only way the tortoise gets ahead is by sticking its neck out. If you want to stay safe inside your boxy shell, then you needn't stick out your neck; but if your life is going to show its promise and vigor, then risk taking is required. The only safety is lifelong involvement. Benjamin Franklin wrote, "He that is secure is not safe." Helen Keller called security "a superstition." To apply these notions to aging, you've got to have guts to grow old.

I am consulted routinely by older patients who seek my

counsel about taking a trip for some celebratory purpose. My invariable advice is to go. I encourage even the frailest of patients to get spruced up, buy the ticket, and enjoy themselves. What's the worst thing that can happen? They might die. Isn't that the way you want to die—after a wedding, graduation, or birth? Similarly, surgery sometimes becomes an issue for my older patients. Rarely, if ever, is age alone a reason not to operate. In fact, it is often safer to operate than not.

Someone wisely observed, "We live too short and die too long." If you accept this premise, what is the best strategy to make it happen? By taking risks. Hunkering down results in protracted decay and dependency. Opportunities for creativity vanish when risk taking is abandoned. Your aging should have as much creativity left in it as possible.

Risk taking means not acceding to time's calendar, because until now our read of the calendar has been wrong. Risk taking means taking a volunteer task or writing your life history at 85, climbing a peak or taking sailing lessons at 80, serving in local government or baby-sitting at 90. Risk taking is buying a pet, establishing a serious new social contact after widowhood, or learning to square dance or waltz, buying bright clothes or a convertible, starting a vegetable garden or housing a graduate student. Risk taking means staying alive until it's over. Risk taking is daring to be 100.

STEP 24. Stay in Control

The importance of maintaining self-efficacy as we age cannot be overstated. It is the heart and soul of successful aging. To age successfully, you must continue to develop your personal resources, and to do this, you must have self-efficacy.

This term "self-efficacy" is not widely used, but essentially it has the same meaning as "control," "coping," "self-sufficiency," "autonomy," or "independence." The opposite of self-efficacy is helplessness or hopelessness. The prescription for self-efficacy is: (1) small steps of mastery, (2) peer examples, (3) social persuasion, and (4) diminishment of failure cues. You may start to lose personal control as you age; nevertheless, you should still keep this prescription prominently in your life.

Taking small steps of mastery means creating minor strategies to offset the clear losses that accompany living a long life. The easy course is to defer to the various negative cues that growing older carry (Every day in every way life is worse). It takes clear vision to offset these cues and assert the opposite attitude, that life can be better despite loss. Creation of such a strategy is not a denial of reality, but rather a deliberate modest effort to establish small platforms of competence. Small steps of mastery mean developing little daily acts of involvement, commitment, and positive risk taking. Being older provides the perspective that makes the shaping of these steps easier. Among the elements of life that can help are family, friendships, hobbies, pets, volunteer work, political courses, and learning.

Peer examples are important, too, for providing inspiration. Keep your antennae tuned to people your age who have learned how to live on the positive side of the ledger of life. Until recently, the legions of wonderfully aged persons have been few and worthy examples rare. But with the new identification of the power and potentials inherent in older people, it will become easier and easier to find examples of people at ages 80, 90, 100, and beyond who will teach you how it's done.

Beyond looking to others as examples, many studies have shown that smart people live longer. You've got to be smart to be old. Most of the new knowledge on aging erases the many negatives handed down to us by those who were not rigorous in their observations. Arm yourself with facts and usable knowledge.

Finally, offset potentially discouraging cues, such as achy legs, fatigue, or slow improvement following loss or illness. A little aspirin or Tylenol helps achy legs; an afternoon nap is strong medicine for fatigue; and development of an optimistic time perspective counteracts the impatience or discouragement after loss. Nature is wonderfully resilient. You are no less.

Self-efficacy is a strong suit of armor as you head across the minefield of life. You should tend it, cherish, and enforce it as your decades accumulate. Stay in charge.

⌐ STEP 25. Maintain the Creative Spark

It is widely reported that imagination and creativity are found most commonly in young people, despite inexperience and lack of perspectives. As you age, then, it is your responsibility to sustain the voltage of your enthusiasm. In the early part of life, you are busy preparing the canvas, tuning the musical instrument, but it is later on that new melodies and fresher images should emerge—if you stay sharp.

The perspective brought by age reveals that life has losses all along the way. But experience allows you to view the bruises and bumps as temporary hurts, which almost always time heals. Recognition of this process contributes to self-renewal and maintenance of the creative spark.

The creative artist seems to have a demon in his or her breast, constantly scratching to command attention. This demon manifests itself as a restlessness and a sense of incompletion. If life is to be truly complete, creative energy must be sustained for the full ten decades.

To write another book, learn a new language, or pursue a different research idea in my 90s is my idea of stretching the creative process. Yours may be to take a watercolor or pottery class, or grow prize orchids.

As a prescription for creativity, continue to saturate, incubate, illuminate, and validate. Seek opportunities to use your unique experience and talent in new ventures. After all, you have more paint in your bucket and notes in your music because you have lived longer. But having the paint and the music isn't enough. You have to pick up the brush or bow and start painting and fiddling. The world will be a brighter place because of the enduring embers turned to flames.

Inspiration and perspiration are a long-acknowledged combination for creativity. Just because you become old is no reason to believe you are no longer capable of working up a good sweat or sparkling with inspiration. Think big and keep it up.

STEP 26. Seek Wisdom

Of the several advantages of becoming old, the chance to become wise looms large. Given the chance to be strong, rich, beautiful, or wise, for me the obvious choice is to gain wisdom.

It is interesting to note that our electronic age devalues wisdom. Information is king—but knowing facts isn't the same as earning wisdom. And don't think wisdom is a simple byproduct of growing old. It has to be carefully developed. Wisdom is a form of expert knowledge about the basic, important matters of life. Wisdom seems to come most naturally to those who plan to learn and learn to plan. There is an interplay between an ongoing accumulation of basic experience and a studied approach to understanding the content and significance of that experience. Wisdom should be the most valuable attainment of your life, and the ability to grow old allows you more time to reach toward that goal.

According to Paul Baltes, there are five dimensions of a genuinely wise person:

1. That person must know a lot; but more importantly, the knowledge must be about things that matter. Knowing a great deal about inconsequential things will not earn many merit badges for wisdom. Instead, know a lot about important things.

2. Know how things work. Know about not just what things are—how big, strong, tall, hot, or cold—but how they operate. Know how things, events, people, and societies function. Anatomy is not enough. Know how the world works.

3. Know how the world works over time. Having a snapshot of places, people, or events at a single moment is not very revealing. Develop an expert knowledge system of how the world works over time.

4. Develop a priority system that allows you to see the world through other people's eyes. Know that what seems important to you at this time may be quite different from what another person from a different time or culture deems significant.

5. Have a tolerance of complexity and ambiguity. Recognize that many situations exist for which there is no ideal solution—only the best for the particular situation—and that the best solution may be different tomorrow.

The individual who has lived long and with direction enough to accumulate these five competencies will be a wise person—a person wonderfully aged and worthy of our admiration.

STEP 27. Be a Responsible Ager

Some time ago, I was a guest on a live talk show on CNN. I was busy beating my breast about how good it feels to be in shape as you age when the host turned to a flamboyant, overstuffed female guest in her studio and asked, "What do you think of what Dr. Bortz just said?" The guest replied, "I don't care a hoot about what the doctor said. Whenever I feel like taking a walk, I lie down. I love the fattest chops I can find. Doctors don't know anything." Then the host turned back to me and asked, "Dr. Bortz, what do you say to that?" I replied, "As an American, I respect the right of any individual to say and do what they want as long as it is responsible. I don't like the idea that our doctors' offices, hospitals, and morgues are filled with people who thumb their noses at commonsense personal health practices and then expect the rest of the world to take care of them, and further yet to pay for it. Rights derive from responsibilities." I shut up, and the show went for a station break.

Millions of hours of thousands of people's time—not to mention tens of billions of our tax dollars—have been spent in an effort to design a system that will administer and pay for our sickness problems more effectively. In my view, there is not enough money in the federal treasury to take care of irresponsible behavior. If someone insists on jumping out of airplanes without a parachute and then expects the doctors and tax-payers to pay for the splatter, we can never have a workable system. Further, we should accept the fact that we will never cure aging, even though the present system insists on trying.

The only sensible system is one that rewards responsible behavior. If I were the health czar, I would seek a system that rates individuals on their health risks just as teenage drivers are rated by insurance companies. If 60 percent of medical encounters are the result of behavioral issues, then these need to be addressed front and center. The concept of health care as a basic human right is fragile in the first place (are food, a home, a car rights?), but if a health problem is the result of a knowing dereliction of self-care, then the idea that it is a right crumbles away instantly.

Previously, we lacked sufficient knowledge to act responsibly, because responsibility ultimately emerges from knowledge. Now we have lived long enough and developed enough valid and documented information on which sound behaviors can be based.

As you grow older, your opportunity and obligation to act responsibly increases. You become less self absorbed and move more toward an integrated view of your personal relationship with the other players in your life. You act more responsibly, and as a result you serve as an example to younger citizens.

STEP 28. Have Options

The newborn has a million doors open to her. The dying person has but one. Life can be thought of as a progressive decrease in the number of options that it presents to you. One of the simple strategies to preserve options is to live a long time. A centenarian by definition will have had many more options available to him or her than will a 40-year-old. So if you want to retain your options, the first rule is to live a long time.

Having options means having freedom. The prisoner's list of options is pretty short; the poet's is infinite. Imagination and optimism are valuable allies in the creation and maintenance of options.

To maintain options is to acknowledge what is possible and deny what is impossible. Options create optimism. It costs energy to maintain options, but increase in freedom and opportunity is well worth the effort. Learning, too, creates options. The smarter you become, the greater will be your options. This means hearing, seeing, sensing, traveling, and experiencing what this big world of yours can offer. It is a rich platter. Your menu is incredibly varied, but you need imagination and energy to pursue and update the menu.

As you age, the tendency is for options to become constricted. You tend to venture less far and keep your windows less open. As a child, your antenna was open to virtually any stimulus that happened by. Some venturings are unpleasant and serve to condition you by avoidance. The trend toward safety and security in aging people limits exposure, and thereby options.

You are not likely to fall down if you are lying down, but you are not going to get anywhere, either. Work toward maintaining, even broadening, your options. Remain as free, open, and risk taking as you were at a younger age, and you will minimize the withering effects of disengagement.

Keeping your options open may mean enacting an active policy of seeking new opportunities. In theory, your options should increase as you age and understand more how the world works and the opportunities it presents. If all you know is your mother's nipple, your vision will remain constricted and your life narrow. You need to stretch your imagination, expand your vistas, enlarge your base of competence and interest and keep as many forks in your road as your energy can allow. The person who has explored the most options has the broadest horizon.

⌐ STEP 29. Be a Good Neighbor

Mark Twain noted that the strongest debit against our intelligence is that we blandly set ourselves up as the "head" animals. Such arrogance has biblical precedent, as Genesis urges us to "subdue nature." Environmental scavenging has been justified on religious grounds, restating dominion over the "fishes of the sea, the fowl of the air, and every living thing that moveth upon the earth."

With hindsight, we can understand the naïveté of the early scribes—we didn't understand the interrelatedness and interdependency of all things bright and beautiful until relatively recently. It is interesting to observe, of course, the much greater nature sensitivity "primitive" cultures have exhibited. We have learned much from them, and we still have more to learn. Buckminster Fuller said, "Nature is trying very hard to make us succeed, but Nature does not depend on us, we are not the only experiment."

First we learned that the universe does not revolve around the Earth. Then we discovered that our modern self is a very recent experiment of nature and our future existence is in no way guaranteed. Many painful lessons of history assert that salvation rests not on arrogance but on understanding and cooperation. The longer you live, the more evident your interdependency with all of nature—with your family and community most obviously, but also with the fish, fowl, and redwoods as well.

We all individually have an ongoing need to reconcile and integrate some sense of personal self with the rest of nature: How do I and the rest of the world work together? We achieve a higher relationship with the world, a consonance, as we react to and respect our environment. The Earth is our house, our common home. Some creatures are known to soil their nests. We seem to be in that group. Sooner or later, however, we will learn. Early in life the preoccupation is with the self. This is energy consuming. As we age, it becomes clear that the world really wasn't created just for us, and the more you turn this proposition around and find a way to help the world, it starts to make better sense. We become integrated.

To be 100 is a cherished destiny, but when you get there you want the earthly house in which you live to be habitable and generous. To exit your world without impact is too modest a goal. It should be better because you were here. Plant a tree, pick up litter, feed the birds, honor nature. It is the only home you have.

_⊓_ **STEP 30.** Cherish Experience

Nothing is so sad as a moment wasted, an opportunity missed, or an experience that is lost. Of all the Earth's resources, human experience is the most in need of recycling. Consider the vast variety of treasures you may accumulate over a lifetime. None is more valuable or unique than experience. It has been won at the cost of thousands of risks taken, wins and losses, expectations denied and affirmed. But sad to say, almost all of us take this richness to our graves.

My awareness of this truism was heightened initially by my wonderful Uncle Walter, for whom I was named. Uncle Walter was my Dad's older brother and the example Dad followed. He entered Jefferson Medical School directly out of high school, graduated with an M.D. at age 23, and then returned to his home in western Pennsylvania to practice medicine for seventy years, until he died at age 94.

As a medical student and young doctor, I loved to spend time with Uncle Walter in the hope that some of his rich patina would rub off on my roughness. He had seen almost everything there was to see in medicine. Our times together were too short, and then he died, and all that richness, unique and wonderful, went with him. Why couldn't he have written it down or recorded in some way his life learning? As Alex Haley wrote, "When an old person dies it is like a small library burning."

I was expressing my personal sense of loss to Nils Nilsson, friend and head of the famous Stanford Computer Science Department. He listened and asked if I had ever heard of the deep-well diggers. I did know about Red Adair, who, with others like him, flew all over the world whenever an urgent occasion required his unusual talent of gauging things thousands of feet below the Earth's surface. Adair and cohorts have a unique competence that has developed not as a result of graduate courses taken or scientific reports read, but as a product of decades of on-the-job experience. They know where an oil field, ore vein, or subterranean lake lies, just because they know. Their precious abilities were quickly recognized by others, who decided to debrief the deep-well diggers in a specific protocol. Much as an astronaut or Indian scout was debriefed after a mission to find out what they had learned, the deep-well diggers were grilled to take full advantage of their knowledge and thereby ensure that their experiences would not be lost to time, as was Uncle Walter's.

What if you had as a life task the obligation to record in writing or otherwise the three things life has taught you? What if, on your 100th birthday, you, with honored ceremony, reveal what you've learned over your lifetime? The expectation of fulfilling this obligation would become a challenge in itself. Alternatively, on a less expansive scale, you can write your life history—who you were at each decade, what you did and what you learned. Why not write your life history for your descendants? Since earliest times, the old were the repositories of knowledge, the keepers of tradition and history, the ones with life perspective. Correspondingly, we should keep a life journal for the last of life.

Each of us should pass on what we have learned through experience, to develop a chain letter of life meaning. In living life fully, learn to pass it on.

STEP 31. Get High on Helping

It's a jungle out there. Every living thing, the beasts and the vines, seems intent on making every effort to achieve every advantage. *Survive* is the basic message. Selfishness is sternly coded on genetic material, which most of nature passes on. For the majority, sympathy is a sentimental illusion. Newborns and young children have little on their minds except their own tightly centered comfort.

But then something happens. We wince at someone else's hurt. We cry at movies. We develop empathy. Scientists are at work trying to find out from which part of our brain this empathy emanates, as well as what influences shape or inhibit it.

It has been shown that degree of selflessness is tightly tied to kin, the implication being that the preservation of the gene pool is paramount to its development. You would sacrifice for a blood relative more readily than for a stranger. Even wartime heroism is identified as sacrifice for those similar to one's self.

It appears that empathy, which may not be common in nature, can be developed in us. To aim for 100 with nobility, you need to identify and search out causes that you feel are important. You need to join an environmental organization, participate in local government, or engage in educational activities. You need to spend more time with people you care about and who care about you. En route, do not assume that the bottom line of your effort is measured in dollars and cents. An exclusively economic life approach is ill fated. The true bottom line of life lies in its contribution.

To develop altruism, a sense of time perspective is important. As you view the world at a given instant, personal survival is given the highest value. But as you begin to view the world as interrelated and reflective of a time dimension, the connectedness to others begins to make sense.

The older you become, the more your empathy has a chance to express itself. The older you become, the less important you as a person are in the total scheme of things. You realize that your importance is only seen in context with others. Time allows you, compels you, to love not just yourself but the others in your world. Pierre Teilhard de Chardin wrote, "Someday we shall harness the energies of love, and then for the second time in the history of the world, man will have discovered fire."

In helping something or someone else to survive, the person who is most likely to benefit is you.

_Γ_ **STEP 32.** Learn to Learn

The brain has been equated with a computer, but to me, the brain is more like an investment account than a computer. The more you use it, the more smarts you will have. That which you learn when you are a child will still be with you when you need it later in life. Intelligence is the great enricher and modulator of the mind. There are multiple types of intelligence: spatial, verbal, musical, self-knowledge, and so on. None is superior to any other. The higher your IQ, the higher is the balance in your brain bank.

Someone once wrote that a good life curriculum would require knowing everything about something and something about everything; therefore, it is reasonable to propose that you can create a lifelong learning investment strategy that will build your best brain. Knowing how long you might live—and then making plans for that duration—requires sound planning. Your formal learning may experience stops in high school, age 18, or college, age 22. This may have been appropriate when you could expect to live only to 45 or so, but what if you live to 100? Have your educational strategies and institutions conformed to this new reality? It is estimated that the knowledge base doubles every eight to ten years. If you read your last book at age 22 and go another 80 years without another effort at learning, it is clear that your contact with the knowledge store will be dysfunctional.

It is clear, too, that information is forming ever faster and greater as time passes. The information superhighway provides a virtually limitless opportunity to stretch your brain. Is your brain up to the task of processing the available information? Do you lose that ability as you age? Some do, but 30 percent of 80-year-olds perform as well as 40-year-olds, who are presumably in their mental prime. Therefore, it's clear learning capacity need not decline with age.

Also helpful are continued life involvements and meaningful experiences. Having an attitude that is flexible and adaptable facilitates late-life learning. Interestingly, individuals involved in long marriages find that their mental abilities tend to converge, with the brighter partner elevating the other's capacity. This is no surprise; cognitive benefits derive from a smart spouse.

There are three basic forms of power: physical, mental and economic. To me mental power has precedence. As the old saw goes, "A fool and his money are soon parted." Money means little to an unenlightened mind. Likewise, brawn without brain is an imbalanced delegation of power. Be a learning machine.

STEP 33. Don't Kill Yourself

The ability to live long consists first of not dying short. Your chance of living to 100 is increased substantially if you don't insist on jumping off a high bridge without a parachute at 30.

Although death certificates say heart attacks, stroke, or cancer, the real cause of death is usually smoking, excessive drinking, stress, a bad diet, or an inactive lifestyle. The usual diagnoses really hide the basic villains. Seventy percent of illness and death is attributable to behaviors that are yours to direct.

Cigarette smoking is under severe indictment as the single most easily identified destructive behavior. Five people die every minute because of smoking. If smokers were required to cover the higher costs of their medical expenditures, every smoker would need to pay an extra $1,500 per year. The terrible tragedies caused by smoking that I alone have witnessed in my medical life are deeply unsettling. To me, smoking cigarettes is like driving through a blinking red light. It gives no warning of its impact until it is too late.

Alcohol comes in second to cigarettes as an addictive villain. The body is so wonderfully forgiving that its tolerance for alcohol is major. For a person to drink enough alcohol to damage the liver, he or she must concentrate on the effort. The main problem of alcohol, therefore, comes not from bodily injury but from the social conflicts that swirl around its use.

Twenty percent of diseases can claim a substantial alcohol component. And as everyone knows, alcohol and gasoline are a dangerous mix; half of traffic fatalities result from this mixture.

How do you know if you have an alcohol problem? There are many guidelines and lists of questions, but a single simple challenge is enough. Who is in charge, you or the alcohol? When you take a drink, are you in total charge of the timing, the amount, and the consequences, or does the alcohol play a controlling role? If you are truly honest in your answer, you can use alcohol responsibly. If not, you need help.

The tragedies that surround cocaine and heroin use are in the newspaper every day, a continuing blight on our society. I have never heard of an addict making 100.

Finally, the havoc our dietary and lifestyle patterns cause is the major barrier most of us face in reaching 100. If you are intent on participating in a destruction derby with your body as the vehicle, no amount of health-system reorienting can make any difference. Life is too precious to be wasted on careless and callous neglect. Live your whole life.

STEP 34. Keep Your Senses Sharp

Your vision, hearing, smell, taste, and touch are your connections to the world. They indicate your relationship with your surroundings. Without them, you would be living in a dark, quiet box.

Many older people tend to withdraw from the world. One of the main strategies to living to be 100 and being vital all the way is to keep your senses tuned and alert to the world. Management of your senses is a major planning step to developing endurance.

It is common knowledge that your senses dull as you age. Ninety percent of people who reach age 90 have some form of cataract. Similarly, the drugs that people take can have their effect on the senses; aspirin affects hearing, for example. If you are to stay engaged for ten decades, you need to be sharp and sensitized. As you lose contact with your environment, your mind tends to wander. Sensory deprivation results in loss of ambition and awareness of yourself in your world.

Routinely, I see older patients who have been brought in by their families because they are losing it. They are functioning poorly and risk dropping out of effective life. One of my first probes is to assess their senses. Often, I identify major deficits and prescribe urgent corrective action. Of course, the tendency is to ascribe the changes to aging alone. The terms "presbyopia" and "presbycusis" (*presby* = old, *opi* = vision, *cusi* = hearing) are heard too often. Doctors assert, "you can't see or hear because you're old." Such attitudes are both wrongheaded and damaging.

Most sensory deficits can be treated. Loss in vision and hearing can be treated successfully. The treatment can be medical, surgical, mechanical, or environmental. Eye drops, cataract surgery, bright lights, and hearing aids are important sense enhancers. It is never too late to improve the senses.

We seem much more conditioned to assuring that our teeth are well tended than our eyes and ears. I suggest that every five years you need an inventory of all your senses, and if you find any of them to be interfering with your quality of life, ask for a referral to an expert.

Life is full of challenges. You need to be able to react with precision, speed, and appropriateness if you are to meet them and channel your energies to your best benefit.

⌐ STEP 35. Train Your Brain

The principal myth about aging concerns the brain. It is commonly assumed that your brain power diminishes with age, but like other dimensions of existence, most of the decline is not due to aging; it is intellectual flab. Like a leg in a cast, when unused the brain deteriorates. Studies have shown that watching television requires less brain energy than looking at a wall. TV is trance enhancing.

When a certain part of the brain is stimulated by a life task, more blood goes to that area. For example, your vision is focused in the back of your brain. When you perform a visual task, the back of the brain receives increased blood flow, and therefore more oxygen and nutrients.

Intellectual challenge and enrichment thereby cause actual structural changes in the brain. It grows, just like your biceps do when you perform chin-ups. The tiny branches of brain cells sprout new branches when the brain is stimulated.

None of this information is in any way surprising. It is just the way nature works. Your structure and function depend on active stimulation for growth and vitality. The natural world has little tolerance for organisms that cease to grow. Your brain is no exception.

It is suggested that Alzheimer's disease affects smart people less. This doesn't mean that smart people don't get Alzheimer's disease, but the theory holds that if you're smart, you'll have a larger mental repertoire to draw from before the deficits caused by Alzheimer's kick in.

But how to train a brain? This is where we need lots of work. Predictably, brain drugs such as certain amino acids emerge to do our brain work for us. No one knows if they might work or not, but I disparage our eternal effort to find shortcuts. We need a brain-exercising program to keep our most meaningful organ brisk and reactive. The details of such a curriculum have not been worked out yet, and it will vary greatly among us, but for starters I suggest we (1) write a letter a day; (2) do volunteer work; (3) learn a language; (4) be physical; (5) stay social; (6) learn to play a musical instrument; (7) be active in government and protecting the environment; (8) care a lot about things; (9) be necessary.

Use your brain. Build your brain.

⌐⌐ **STEP 36.** Build Memory

It is more important to forget than it is to remember. If we remembered even 10 percent of all the information we receive, we would be in a lot of trouble. The Greeks used to think of the brain of children as an empty slate on which the experiences of a lifetime were accumulated. Just imagine the mess that would occur if everything you heard, saw, felt, smelled, tasted, and learned was crowded onto that blackboard. You need an efficient eraser to live effectively.

How often do you or others complain that they remember too much? It is usually the opposite complaint. It is said that memory loss is one of the inevitable consequences of growing old, and it is, somewhat. A young person can recall an average of eight or ten nouns on a list; older persons six to eight. Yet if you train the older person, she can learn to recall thirty to forty nouns. Of course, if you train a younger person, he will again outperform the older student, but the central point is that training brings gain, and this gain is much greater than the loss that time alone conveys.

There are essentially two types of memory, short and long. Short-term memories are ones you use for mandatory tasks, like remembering a phone number when it is given to you—but you'll quickly forget it if it is not rehearsed and banked into your long-term memory drawer, where the traces of our important information are stored. Memory is said to have three components: registering, retaining, and retrieving. Registering means coding the event, place, or name into the short-term bank by focusing intently on the effort of remembering. With frenzy or distraction, the coding won't register. Retaining requires rehearsal to secure the item in long-term memory. Retrieval involves recall and recognition. The richer the network from which recall and recognition can be extracted, the better the memory will be.

We know a little bit about improving memory, but we know a lot about what makes it worse. The most prominent threat to our memory is Alzheimer's disease, which robs millions of people of their mental and emotional treasures, but high blood pressure, depression, and many other diseases also rob us of our hard-won intellectual heritage. Numerous drugs, particularly alcohol, blunt our ability to remember.

To reach for 100 requires the creation and retention of a rich lifetime's worth of experiences. You need your memory to record your good and bad efforts. It gives you the opportunity to make enlightened choices, which is what life is all about in the first place.

⌐ STEP 37. Keep Order

When 1,200 centenarians were surveyed to find out their secret to longevity, 90 percent of the group identified the role of order in their lives. Orderliness—not money, not genetics, not health—led the list of beneficial aptitudes. On the face of it, this element seems to lack much emotional or even intellectual appeal. I couldn't envision, for example, a National Association for the Advancement of Order. But the more I read and understand, the more compelling the idea of maintaining order becomes. We know that married people live longer, that adverse life events prejudice longevity, that physical and mental disorders are risk factors.

Order means health. Health means order. Order means the maintaining of the best form and function. A fit body is in perfect order, maintained so by an energy flow. A frail limb or body has low order. It doesn't work well, it needs a transfusion of energy. Growth and adaptability cannot occur without the ordering effect of an energy flow on matter.

How can you translate the need for order into practical guidelines? First, keep moving. Most of the body serves movement purposes, and by using the muscles and bones and joints and tendons for their purposes, their form and function will be assured.

Second, keep learning. For the brain, challenge is as essential as movement is for the muscles. Learning should not be confined to the first two decades of life. New research clearly shows that the used brain gathers no rust. Further, lifelong learning carries with it the joy of seeing. The more complex a thing is, the more orderly it is—like a rainforest. Complex things have many supporting elements that maintain a high order of function. Unlike machines, which seem to malfunction in direct proportion to the number of parts, your body—and particularly your brain—is healthier the more complex and well used it is.

Third, keep the emotions cool. When anger, anxiety, or depression surge beyond a controllable margin, they place your emotional self at risk. "Everything in moderation" has been the rule for thousands of years—moderate temper as well. An angry behavior type is not good for the angry person's health, or anyone else's, either.

Fourth, keep the senses sharp. The senses are your antennae to the world and need to be able to receive the latest relevant information from your environment. The older you become, the more important your senses are to your effective survival.

Fifth, maintain tradition. Time is an honored teacher, and knowledge of personal and community tradition is a valuable memory. Recalling how certain dates and occasions have been celebrated in the past brings increased significance and self-sufficiency. The older you become, the more important your role in maintaining the archives of shared experiences is. Accumulated experience leads to wisdom, and the old are the precious landlords of the home where wisdom lives.

Sixth, renew yourself. One of the great glories of life is its almost infinite capacity for renewal. Renewal means reordering, regrouping. If retreat and disengagement is met by a process of enlightened renewal, then order is recaptured and vigor reasserted. You are never too old to renew.

Order emerges, then, as a central marker of successful aging. Order is not the exclusive domain of theoretical physicists; it is, in fact, the keystone of being a centenarian.

⌐ STEP 38. Be Attractive

The reason women live longer than men is that they usually dress like they are going to a party—unlike men, who always look like they are headed for a funeral. If you want to be 100, be bright, pretty, and clean. Keep a sparkle in your eye and in your step. Keep your hair neat and groomed. Be well shaved. Keep your teeth in good shape, and maintain good hygiene. Nothing is as much of a turnoff as another person who doesn't smell good. Be slim. Be strong. Become buddies with your barber or hairdresser. A hot shower makes anyone feel decades younger.

Dress well. Keep your clothes tidy and tended. The gravy-on-the-tie look doesn't work at any age, but it serves to emphasize images of decay and deterioration. Old clothes are okay if they are not tattered, but it is important to buy new things every so often. The fashion gurus would like you to believe that clothes create your persona. It may be a sales pitch, but nevertheless, your self-image is determined to a fair degree by the type of threads you drape around your body. Despite my suggestions, however, don't use clothes as a disguise. Let yourself show.

Skin sags as you grow older. Loss of elasticity is one of the real markers of aging. The skin on an older person's back of the hand takes longer to snap back than a younger person's. This lack of elasticity causes wrinkles and sagging skin, eyelids, and breasts. For most of us, these wrinkles are merit badges, which we have worked hard to earn. I find older people's faces attractive and much more interesting than those of younger people, which have not yet been etched by life experience. Those canvases have not yet been painted on. Many, however, find the wrinkles a discredit rather than a credit. The 85-year-old mother of one of my colleagues approached me several years ago to ask my opinion about her having a facelift. She certainly didn't need my blessing for this, but I did tell her that facelifts usually last only ten years, so by age 95 she'd probably want another. That fact did not deter her at all.

Attractiveness represents the average—not too big or too small, short or tall, average nose, eye, and lip size—all tied to a gently implied breeding desirability. Health and vigor are inherent. As you age, the reproductive-capacity desirability becomes irrelevant, but the residue of the message of healthfulness and attractiveness remains. Naturally, you want to be around others who radiate good feelings and optimism.

As you reach to 100, you need to keep your trousers pleated, your shoes shined, your hair neatly coiffed, and your smile always ready.

⌐ STEP 39. Recognize That Sex Is for Life

Is sex after 50 an unnatural act, a vestigial remnant designed by nature only for those of reproductive age? Or is sex a life-quality issue, a central function to be protected and cherished, like breathing or eating? Sex is very close to the essence of life. Some biologists claim that it is all there is to life.

Of all your vital functions, sex is the most secret and hidden from the world, but even sadder, it's likely hidden from yourself. Freud made quite a name for himself teaching us how all of us repress our basic sexuality. No one is more repressed than older people. This repression is unhealthy, unnecessary, and just plain dumb. Masters and Johnson, our most esteemed sexologists, assert that education is the key. As we learn more about sexuality across the lifespan, we will become newly able to redefine our own potentials as we age.

The entire field of gerontology is full of myth, and nowhere is the mythology more prevalent than in the area of sex. The first and most pervading myth concerns the reality of sex after 50. The truth is that old people can. Old people do. Old people are sexier than younger people perceive them to be and are sexier than they perceive themselves to be.

I don't mean to say that old people can and do have sex the same way as they did at age 20. What is the same at 70 as it is at 20? You're wrong to try to compare yourself to yourself fifty years ago; instead, try to look at others your same age. Here is where the ignorance quotient is very high.

Until recently sexual inadequacy in older people was presumed to be largely psychological. Now we know that there may be a number of physical issues as well, illness and drug use among them. In fact, most sexual problems in older people are physical. For men, they involve potency issues; for women, opportunity. Both men and women must give themselves permission to remain sexual. Older people of both sexes must realize that sex is not just okay to think about and preserve, but a major positive life force. The famous idiom "Use it or lose it" echoes again and again.

A key feature of sexuality is responsibility. Much of the negative imagery that surrounds sex in general derives from a widely broadcast lack of respect for others and even for oneself when the juices start to flow. As you age, this issue should become less and less relevant. Bonding and intimacy, if they are to be the positive life forces they should be, demand easy communication and constant mutual trust.

A robust sex life into the 90s and beyond is the ideal. All it needs is guts and smarts. Smarts is the knowledge that the source of self-identity and glory can be ours the whole way, and guts the courage to keep sex free and romantic, new and healthy.

Alex Comfort wrote that having sex is like riding a bicycle. It takes a bit of energy and a bit of balance, is good for you, and is a hell of a lot of fun.

⌐ **STEP 40.** Stay in Touch

No man or woman is an island. No one stands alone. The evidence for the importance of intimacy in childhood is clear. One of the major risks of late-life institutionalization is the loss of the opportunity to give and receive intimacy, and the loss of opportunity for intimacy is the supreme disengagement and the risk of true dependency. Connectedness is not only necessary at the start of life, but at the end as well. Studies have shown that connected people have less than half the mortality rates as lonely people, and the closer the relationship, the more powerful the survival effect.

Living alone is bad for your heart, bad for your immunity, bad for your mind. The key to keeping laboratory rats alive is not nutritional nor medical care, but the simple availability of TLC. Old rats live substantially longer merely because they are caressed. It sounds good to me.

As a physician, I identify the power of touching. I have a number of patients in nursing homes. Many of their circumstances are pretty forlorn. As "untouchable" as they appear, however, I make it a standard practice to touch them, even those who seem insensitive or hostile. I don't know if it helps them, but I feel sure it helps me. President Reagan recalls the nurse who held his hand after he was shot. "Her holding my hand as I was lying there with this bullet in my chest helped save my life." The presence of a friendly face—and touch—in the aseptic environment of emergency rooms and intensive care units is an unexplored force.

A touch agenda reveals five different varieties across the spectrum of intensity: (1) functional; (2) social; (3) friendly; (4) sensate; and (5) sexual. We need all five, but problems arise as to when and how to administer and receive. As with other human connectedness, the stimulus needs to be appropriate for the giver and the receiver. And as we need to learn how to touch, we also need to learn how to be touched. Too many of us are touch averse. At the extreme, this leads to disengagement: "Leave me alone! Don't touch me!" At a lesser extreme is the more common tendency to avoid situations in which touch is likely to occur. Touching someone and being touched is somewhat risky. It involves a sort of contact, and the mutuality of the contact is critical. As you grow older intelligently, you must remember and integrate the importance of touch. For much of nature, touch is a survival tool—in all likelihood it is for you as well.

One of the principal barriers to touching and intimacy as we age is the discordance between male and female lifespans. Most married women are widowed for eight-plus years at the end of their lives. What are we supposed to do about this as yet inadequately explained gap in the average ages of death of men and women? We men are going to have to do a better job of addressing this major shortfall (mainly by staying healthy into old age).

"Touch hunger" and "intimacy starvation" are major issues for us if we dare to be 100. Hug, caress, nuzzle, stroke, rub, pet, stay in touch. This advice is better medicine than anything I have in my black bag.

⌐⌐ STEP 41. Take RX Pet

The Sioux chant goes, "I sing for the animals."

What would our world be like if we were the only animals in it? If there were no robins, no porpoises, no spiders, no tigers, no frogs, no eagles, no bears, no butterflies, no dogs? What a lonely and sad planet it would be. Animals are part of our family. They give so much to us in millions of ways.

Pets are wonderful for people of any age, but they are of

particular significance to older people. They often become an older person's surrogate family. Early in life most of us have the happy bonds of family members to nourish and sustain. As we age, our families fragment, and too often a lone elder remains behind. Enter the pet. A newly widowed 74-year-old can derive great benefit from an animal companion. A nursing home is a logical site for an animal presence. The type of pet an individual chooses can be imaginative—beyond the standard dog and cat—to include tropical fish, birds, deer, squirrels and rabbits, even ferrets or snakes. Having a pet commits us to caring about something outside ourselves. It means being responsible for another's wants and needs. Such a relationship between human and animal grows only with a generous spirit.

Yet the value of a relationship with an animal, like anything else in life, is directly proportional to the energy and care that you invest in it. If you are willing to learn and show mutual respect, pets can teach you much about life. Observance of a pet's life cycle helps you understand your own life phases better. Experiencing a pet's death helps you understand your own mortality. Pet grief is an intense human experience, and the sense of loss must be factored into your menu of life events.

The existence of the strong emotional bonding between humans and pets has led to innumerable efforts to use animals as therapy for a wide assortment of human hurts. Scratching your dog's ears not only lowers the dog's pulse rate and blood pressure, but yours as well. Patients who have had a heart attack and also have a pet have an easier recuperation than those who lack a pet. Control of diabetes is improved if there is an animal in the house. Both survival of cancer and recovery after surgery are aided by relationships with an animal friend.

Pets are wonderful antidepressants. How could any depression survive the joy and enthusiasm of a golden retriever puppy? Similarly, neurologically impaired people seem to find that pets provide strong assistance in helping them overcome their limitations. The intimacy of a soft head, a warm tongue, and a wagging tail is strong medicine indeed.

In the final analysis, a pet is a fine doctor and a dear friend.

⌐ STEP 42. Keep Family Strong

The family is the moral anchor. It is within the family structure that we first learn our values. All of us start life in a family context—many fewer end life that way. Something has gotten lost along the way. In family relationships, you move beyond being a lone individual. Family helps you solve problems, share stress, and develop common defenses. In theory, your relationship with the changing personalities in your life should become richer as you traverse life's stages. As children, we are receivers of energy from our parents. As you live, your role shifts from receiving to giving energy. The older you become, the more you should have to give. Of course, society doesn't always recognize this contribution.

Biologists teach that you maintain attachment and devotion in direct proportion to shared genetic material—that familial connection makes survival sense—and you construct your life strategies to share the common goal of family survival. With the sharing of goals, win-win propositions arise— a "one for all and all for one" attitude. Relationship skills within the family are developed, relationship skills that will help in interactions with the rest of the world. In this sense, the family unit becomes the rehearsal hall for the theater of life. The negotiations and problem solving that occur among family members involve the same skills as are necessary in the workplace, and the world community at large.

Of course, the family does not exist in isolation. The family unit lives in its own social environment, just as every individual does. Development of shared resources and coping capacity allow for collective strengths that no single individual can muster. The nest serves you admirably as the first home, but no one can stretch your wings for you. That responsibility belongs to you alone. Successful growth implies a simultaneous development of individual strength and preservation of the family context.

In this accelerating world, family life is an option—not a necessity. Change in the social environment, particularly the opening of the workplace to women, has splintered traditional models. Single-parent families are distressingly common. I retain my conviction that individual growth and development occurs best in two-parent households. Continuity of relationships is exempted in the single-parent family. Disorder prevails.

Ordered structures require a constant supply of energy to sustain them. The family is no different. The common premise is that the family is so natural that it more or less takes care of itself. Not so. It must be carefully and enthusiastically nurtured.

One of the elements in preserving the integrity of the family is the reestablishment of the role of the older members in the functional unit. Too often the older family members—grandfather, grandmother, and others—are useless vestiges, confused in their roles. The younger generations don't know what their role is, either. The existence of four-generation families is increasingly common. The second from the bottom, commonly termed the "sandwich" generation, becomes the vital center; the other three are dependent on this center. This structure is not normal and cannot functionally be sustained. The two older generations need to affirm their continued responsibilities and rehearse their future roles early in life. In her 90s my mother was embarrassed, because she didn't know how to react with my children and their children—she hadn't, after all, expected to live this long. You, however, should expect to become grandparents and great-grandparents and plan correspondingly for your integrating role in the evolving family.

Older people have more time to listen, fewer personal urgencies, an increased sense of context. They are the family archivists. The older members are the family prophets, the signposts that show where the young may or may not go. As you reach toward 100, your family opportunities and responsibilities should shift, yet endure. The success of our culture, and the quality of our lives, is heavily dependent on our respect for, and nurturing of, our family.

⌐⌐ STEP 43. Don't Take Yourself So Seriously

My dad used to ask, "Who's going to remember a hundred years from now?" This simple nugget of wisdom has helped me through a thousand mini-crises—situations I thought had doom written all over them but were in reality only small blips on the big screen of a lifetime. Such perspective is yet another advantage of growing older.

The world, of course, is the way it is; it is therefore the way in which we perceive it that is critical. Norman Cousins delighted in the discussion of positive emotions. Several years ago I arranged a whole-day meeting of six hot-shot neurochemists with Norman. We assembled at the Behavioral Science Center at Stanford. For hours, the scientists described the elegant new brain studies of depression, anger, anxiety. Norman said nothing until near our adjournment. "But don't you feel that the positive emotions of love, caring, purposefulness have equivalent but opposite effects on the brain?" The individuals of the assemblage blinked, and quietly nodded assent. There are no studies on what can go right—only on what can go wrong.

Every one of us knows the value of laughter—Norman used to call it "internal jogging"—and the field of humor has been subjected to scientific analysis. Our endorphins go up when Jonathan Winters, Bill Cosby, or Robin Williams comes on the TV screen. Our immune response improves. Humor seems to derive out of an unusual, unexpected combination. In its best form it allows us to comment on the jumbled concepts and absurdities of our existence. It allows flexibility and plasticity and prevents us from rigidity of thought and perspective.

Often a patient enters my office with enough complaints to last forty years. In itself, the length of the list is a tipoff. I listen as dutifully as I am able and frequently comment, "No one among us is healthy enough to withstand such self-scrutiny as you exhibit. If any us were to hold a magnifying mirror to ourselves and preoccupy ourselves with the analysis that such an examination would inevitably reveal, we'd all have a list such as yours." Health and humor connote lack of self-consciousness and an active reciprocation with the rest of the world. Tolerance is a cousin to good humor. Good humor is never cruel. If it hurts, it is not humor.

Humor can detoxify not only medical illness, but it can also be used as an approach to problem solving on numerous levels. Political impasses, family discords, and business disagreements can all be solved by the appropriate humorous analogy. Less posturing and less pontificating—and more generosity of spirit—bring troubles of all sorts into clearer focus and order.

No one is ever too old to forget the Magic Kingdom. Fairy tales are never far beneath our surface. Clowns probably do as much good as doctors in providing relief and understanding. No day can be all bad if it produced a laugh.

To plan for 100 years does not mean, however, using humor as a silly retreat from reality. The older you become, the more able you should be to abstract yourself from the inane and meaningless and find delight and positive energy in the unexpected and discontinuous. Surprise parties are fun because of their very unpredictability. When each day is predictable, life is boring.

Someone observed that the size of your funeral depends on the weather. Wear a costume to your funeral; make someone else happy.

Make your last thought a happy one.

STEP 44. Work with Stress

Stress is acknowledged as being an active partner in many of the diseases making the rounds at hospitals and doctors' offices. The chart may read heart problems or stroke, but the real culprit is often stress.

The speed and complexity of modern life seems wonderfully suited to producing stress. The high "event density" of daily existence is a rat-a-tat bombardment to the nervous system.

Stress is much more than just time and change. More important than the event that causes the stress is how each of us reacts to it. Some people can walk through a field of wasps and never break stride. For others, a mosquito in the same county elicits great anxiety. Any life of value will have bucketsful of potential stress producers; the secret to stress is to welcome it, work with it, and use its energy and challenges to make your life better. A Gallup poll of Fortune 500 top executives found that 60 percent of them found stress to be exhilarating and creative.

The most central ingredient in building a familiarity with dealing with stress is perspective. If you view every miniature departure from the routine as a threat of major consequence, then you're in for tough going. Stress expert Dr. Robert Eliot advises two things: "First, don't sweat the little things, and second, everything is a little thing." It is always a kick to think back a year or so and identify the things that were keeping us awake at night. Almost invariably, they have melted into non-significance.

Other stress antidotes are good—strong health and a positive outlook counteract stress. It is important, too, to look stress in the eye. Pretending that a big bill, an overdue doctor's or dental visit, or a family conflict doesn't exist makes resolution very tough. Relaxation skills and a sense of humor help. Exercise is also a terrific stress reducer.

One excellent way to counteract stress is to allow yourself to grow old. As you age, you'll find the seemingly unsurmountable problems of your youth pretty shallow. Aging brings perspective that only time and experience can provide. Ultimately, growing older is a solvent into which early life stresses dissolve.

◻ STEP 45. Have Time Sense

Suicide Prevention's motto, "Suicide is a permanent solution to a temporary problem" puts time into an important perspective. The hopelessness of the moment and the rush for immediate gratification are connected to no time dimension. The Now Generation consumes itself and its time and hence it has either no or few tomorrows to anticipate. We are paying all a price for this lack of time sense.

The likelihood today of a longer lifespan makes it imperative to understand time. If you are to die at 20 or 40, longitudinal life forces do not have a chance to assert themselves. Gifts of age are real and important, but they can only be achieved by putting in time. Elsewhere in this book I write of the central role time plays in creativity. So, too, does time affect learning, experience, and wisdom, all central themes of the successful life. The process of sequential thought particularly brings power to the enlightened person.

The effect of life choices takes time to become apparent. A fit body or a fit mind grows old at the rate of ½ percent per year. That is slow. Comparatively speaking, an unfit body and mind decays at 2 percent per year—still not a very fast rate—but when you multiply these small differences between 2 percent and ½ percent per year times 30 or 40 years, the short-term variance is magnified many times over.

Research studies on aging are hindered by such lack of time appreciation. Any effort to improve the life quality of old people is expected to work fast—and cheaply. Unfortunately, the deficits that have accumulated over decades are of a different type than, for instance, an individual stepping on a tack. But aging experiments take a long time to conduct, and the results are modest. The quick fix doesn't generally apply to problems that occur late in life. This fact should not, however, provide an excuse for not making the effort. Age is *never* an excuse for not trying. It is never too late. Gian Carlo Menotti says the concept of hell is feeling like you are "too late."

The ability to plan for a whole lifetime is critical. You need both short- and long-term goals. What are you going to be at age 90? The answer depends on planning and confidence that this distant age is not just possible, but probable.

Your ability to predict and manage your fortunes depend in large measure on the competence you have built over decades of life experience. Time allows this development to occur and by itself facilitates success, but only you have the smarts to use this gift. Time should not be the enemy; it should be a major ally. You need to understand it and use it for your best purposes. Time marches on; let us walk in step with it.

⎍ STEP 46. Know Your Primary Doctor

To find the best doctor in town, get out the phone directory and look up your own number. That is the number to call for the best doctor in town—for you. What I mean is that the best healer is within your own skin. Certainly, the medical system stands ready for all sort of heroic miracles, but for the great majority of ailments, self-diagnosis and treatment should be the first plan of action.

Fortunately, there are a number of self-help books available to serve as your textbooks and references. Some of the best are Vickery and Fries's *Take Care of Yourself, The AMA Manual on Self-Care,* and *Healthwise for Life*. Despite a diligent self-diagnosis, however, everyone should have a primary-care doctor, usually a general internist or a family practitioner. Primary physicians are broadly based and can handle 90 percent of medical problems. They also know when and why to refer you to a specialist.

Be an active patient. Your participation is important in your health. Your doctor is not the boss; you are partners in maintaining your well-being. Your ability to communicate with your doctor is also essential. On your first visit to a prospective new doctor, assess whether he or she shares your commitment to health promotion. The physician who becomes interested only when you are sick is a bad choice. Does the physician stay reasonably on time, return phone calls promptly, give adequate/courteous explanations? Is he or she available? You may choose the biggest name in town, but if the name is not on the other end of the phone when you call, what good is the name? Not all good docs make house calls, but any Board-certified doc who does is a good choice. Does your doctor prescribe pills first, or try instead to solve your problem by suggesting other caring strategies? A pill should be the last—and not the first—resort. Getting to know the nurse is also a good step. You will know the doctor better when you have a good relationship with the lady (or gentleman) in white. Ask about tests and medicines, understand recommendations and diagnoses, be aware of costs, and ask "How much?"

Writing questions down before a visit—and then writing down your summary of the visit—is helpful in shaping the value of a medical encounter and its outcome. If you don't understand something after you leave the office, call again and ask. Generally, we are afraid of what we don't understand. A few simple questions can make a big difference in clearing up uncertainties.

Albert Schweitzer wrote, "Each patient carries his own doctor inside of him." We are at our best when the doctor who lives within us has the chance to go to work. When you work together with your doctor, your health is in the best hands.

STEP 47. Pamper Your Glands

Whenever I write a prescription, I feel a pang. I feel I should be able to address the problem in a more natural way. Of course, prescribing a drug is easier, and it takes much less time to write a prescription than it does to investigate what dietary, exercise, or stress-altering strategies are more appropriate.

Prescribing female hormones is an exception, however. I am a firm believer in the strong benefits derived from taking estrogen. In a sense, hormones aren't drugs; taking them replenishes the body's supply of something it has produced for roughly four decades but stopped providing around the middle of life. It is somewhat like giving insulin to a diabetic, to repair an obvious lack of a normally occurring substance.

The main benefit that estrogen provides to older women is its protection against heart and artery disease. With the exception of smokers, premenopausal women are virtually immune to heart problems. But after menopause, heart problems in women start to catch up with those in men as their cholesterol rises. Estrogen promotes higher levels of the good HDL cholesterol, and hormone replacement therapy is generally agreed upon to be good for preventing heart disease.

The second major benefit of estrogens is the protection against osteoporosis. The epidemic of fractures due to weak bones, 1.2 million per year, is to a large degree attributable to a lack of estrogen. This issue is particularly critical for women who have had their ovaries removed early in life; they are at severe risk for osteoporosis.

In the past few months, a third major benefit of estrogen has emerged. It has been shown that the incidence of Alzheimer's disease is lower in women who have taken estrogen. The mechanism for this connection is not yet clear, although the sex hormones have been known for a long time to have effects on brain development.

Like everything else in life, taking estrogen is a mixed blessing. An increased risk of cancers of the uterus and breast has been reported in women undergoing hormone replacement. My suspicion, however, is that much of this increase has resulted from overzealous use of the hormones. Some doctors have unintentionally prescribed doses higher than the norm. To offset this effect, most gynecologists advise the simultaneous use of progesterone, the other ovarian hormone. In turn, the problem with this strategy is that progesterone offsets some of the protective effect of the estrogen. The medical community is still working on combinations that limit the downside of progesterone, such as using it only every third month, for example.

Other side effects of hormone use, including fluid retention and clot-forming tendencies, must be individually approached. All other things being equal, though, I still say go for the estrogen.

So if estrogen is good for women, is testosterone good for men? Although testosterone levels fall with aging, they do not do so to the degree that estrogen does. Also, testosterone stimulates the prostate, which is already a major nuisance to the aging male. We simply need more information before widespread prescription of testosterone can be deemed appropriate.

Hormones matter—a lot. You should exploit their use as you can, but attention to diet, attitude, renewal, and exercise should still hold precedence. If they can help you, though, embrace hormone replacement as part of your DARE to Be 100 plan.

STEP 48. Be a Good Loser

As a young boy, I hated to lose. I threw tons of tantrums when my team lost or my older relatives beat me in gin rummy. Somewhere along the way, though, I grew up. Losses still hurt, but time has taught that the sun will still come up tomorrow. Once again, time lends perspective.

Development during any life period reflects the dynamic interplay between gains and losses. This dynamic brings a less positive balance as we age. Aging does bring losses, inevitably. You simply have to know that every day a little water spills out of your cup. But is the cup partially empty or partially full? If you see it as emptying all the time, it is possible to fall victim to helplessness and hopelessness. The antidote for this attitude is learned hope. It can be taught and learned. When hope perishes, all is lost. Ellen Langer wrote, "There are no failures, only ineffective solutions."

Humor, too, is a tool to use in confronting loss. When we can laugh at defeat, we see its context. We are mindful of the setting. Death is used by some as an excuse for a hell of a party. In my judgment, death, the final loss, hurts for three reasons, but two of them can be dealt with. The first thing that hurts about death is its timing. Almost always it comes too soon. The death of any young person always hurts badly, because it is out of sync with what ought to be. On a personal level, you can avoid this hurt simply by deciding to live long—and then succeeding. The second hurt is the way we die, often without control and dignity. This, too, is approachable and correctable. The third hurt of death is the simple animal sense of loss. But if the first two hurts can be addressed (as in my mother's case; she died healthy at 95), the last loss can be made to feel almost good. Certainly, no matter what, death is a major life passage, but it's more acceptable when it can be turned around and used as a moment for growth, rather than diminishment.

The older you are, the smarter and more experienced you become. Your tolerance of loss is greater, and your ability to reshape the losses holds the opportunity for a more stable and effective life.

One of my most important strengths is a line from a poem that my father adapted from Robert Browning: "Then welcome each rebuff that turns Earth's smoothness rough, that bids each man not sit nor stand but go." This exhortation has been brilliantly powerful for me. It has brought success from many seeming failures. Perhaps I am still a poor loser, but now I use the energy of the loss to promote winning.

STEP 49. Stay in Tune

What do Florence Nightingale, Plato, the drummer for the Grateful Dead, a 90-year-old nursing home resident, and Dr. Oliver Sacks have in common? Answer: They all prescribe music as therapy.

The healing power of music has been recognized for centuries. As Congreave wrote in 1697, "Music has chance to soothe a savage breast, to soften rocks, or bend a knotted oak." Conferences are now devoted to the healing abilities that music offers. Childbirth, tooth extraction, depression, anxiety, compulsion, hypertension, and many other medical conditions are eased by the effects of music. Music can inspire, stir passion, and create intimacy. For every mood there is a form of music, from funeral marches to hard rock. Music is like sex. It reaches deep inside you, and gives you great pleasure.

Music represents the recapture of the maternal heartbeat first heard before birth. The thump and throb is heard in nature's drumbeat. A movie or a TV show without music is a bland experience. Correspondingly, life without music seems one-dimensional, like living only in black and white. Music brings order to life, making sense of a chaotic world and bringing enchantment to silent periods. It makes rich harmonies out of the dissonance all around us. It helps us survive.

What happens to musical encounters as we age? Too often the weariness of old age inhibits the aesthetic opportunities that music and art provide. The weariness is compounded by sensory loss and other functional impairments, which can restrict access to the exhilarating opportunities that permeated early life. As you age, if you disengage from these cherished habits, life becomes merely a pale shadow of its real image.

Concerts, parades, and festivals are integral to living a full life. Make them as much a part of the latter part of life as the earlier part. Sustain your connection to the sound of music. It will, in turn, sustain you.

STEP 50. Stay on the Road

For better or worse, Americans live to drive. Our cars often seem to be more important to us than our homes. For many of us, our legs are just vestigial remnants. It's our cars that keep us moving.

As you age, your car sometimes causes problems. It is both expensive and complicated. I have not yet read of a car maker who designs an age-friendly car. To the contrary, all the ads are pitched to the swift and brassy youth, but a great, great number of gray heads are on the roads, both because they have to be and because they want to be.

Drivers in their 60s average four crashes per million miles. In their 80s that figure rises to fifteen per million miles, still only half the rate of teenagers. Older drivers drive more slowly. A whole slew of reports indicate that older people are safer drivers, and insurance companies know this fact. The periodic drivers' tests imposed by the state motor vehicle department seek to assure our continued competence on the roads. A clear issue is vision, and obviously we need to see to drive or do almost anything else. But what about reflexes and judgment?

Every so often, a family member will call me and express concern that Ma or Pa doesn't seem to be strong enough to continue to drive. This is always a tough one for me, because driving is a mark of independence, and when the ability to drive is restricted, life takes on a new and usually diminished meaning. In many cases, loss of driving privileges might mean loss of an entire repertoire of competency. My first reaction to such a call is to try to learn the facts. How well does he or she see, how vigorous are they, how is their judgment, and what does driving mean to them? Having gone through this exercise, occasionally I find myself stuck. The older person shouldn't drive but still adamantly asserts his or her intent to do so.

My next move is to insist on an objective test, perhaps through one of the local automobile clubs or driving schools. If the individual passes, then everyone is happy. If he is marginal, then he can take driving classes to sharpen his skills. If he fails, then he cannot drive. Sometimes individuals can obtain conditional licenses, which allow them to drive only during the daytime, or on roads with a forty-mile-per-hour or lower speed limit.

Denial of driving privileges can be tempered by various creative strategies. Perhaps a younger family member would agree to drive an older relative in exchange for greater car privileges. Maybe an old pal could provide both wheels and social contact. Finally, a renewed emphasis on walking wouldn't hurt.

For most of you, however, I suggest you keep your driving skills honed, just like everything else you do. Your senses, muscles, and memory all need active tending. Similarly, driving is so important that you need to be sure that your skill at it is not lost as you age.

_⌐_ **STEP 51.** Recognize Depression

For millions, depression is a sullen partner. In all likelihood, many people are depressed at some time or another, but for far too many, the later years are painted in dark blue.

Life gives us lots of things to be depressed about. Nevertheless, events are not the main ingredients for depression. If you let yourself think that life is going to be hard, no matter what anyone says, it's going to be hard. More important than the injuries and insults is how you react to them. If you view life's losses for what they are and learn lessons from them that brace you for the next loss, then similarly, depression recedes. If, however, helplessness and hopelessness result from the perception that being alive means unremitting suffering and that struggle is useless, then depression looms.

Major changes in brain chemistry accompany depression. This is where antidepressant medicines come in. The use of antidepressant medicine for the depressed person is like the use of insulin for a diabetic—it's an effort to repair a chemical deficiency, and it works! But before quickly resorting to the prescription pad, I have always advocated physical exercise as the first line of defense—or maybe offense. As an antidepressant, exercise has sturdy credentials. Each bout of sweating is accompanied by a surge in the production of body molecules called catecholamines, commonly known as adrenaline. These same compounds are not found in abundance in the nervous systems of depressed people.

Exercise, too, has been shown to raise the levels of the upper-compound endorphins, which accompany euphoria and immunize against pain. These endorphins are probably behind the acknowledged addictive quality of exercise.

In taking care of depressed older patients, I try to bring an activist approach. Older people may actually have the advantage over younger people when it comes to depression, because they have broader experience, have taken the lightning hits that every life provides, and understand that time is a wonderful bandage. As I recall the dozens of people over 100 for whom I have cared, I cannot recall a single one who was depressed. Instead, in each case a sense of confidence prevailed.

Perspective is crucial in determining how you take your lumps. There are strong strategies you can develop that help offset depression. Optimism, a sense of humor, and physical fitness are safe, cheap, and universally available techniques. If exploring these options does not lift the burden of depression, ask for help.

⌐┌ STEP 52. Die Well

"I am not afraid of dying," Woody Allen said, "I just don't want to be there when it happens." It would be interesting if we could ask or pay someone else to do it for us, but I don't really know how to approach this proposition.

Most people die in the hospital. For most, this is not necessary—it just happens because of our collective inability to arrange to die at home. A good and decent death has three components—no pain, no tubes, and no loneliness. When these three criteria are satisfied, Woody Allen and the rest of us should have few complaints about our final exit.

Death is rarely characterized by pain that is not manageable. I surveyed the terminal trajectories of the ninety-seven patients in my practice who died in 1989. I analyzed their abilities to move, think, and toilet, and whether they had pain at the end of their lives. Only four did, and it was easily managed.

Tubes are a related issue. Modern medicine couldn't get

along without all the tubes at its disposal, but these should be very carefully used. Tubes are often extremely valuable for acute situations, but they almost never need to be used for long. It is hard to have a life of high quality when tubes are involved.

Loneliness as an accompaniment to death is a social issue that goes way beyond medicine. Someone said that "old age is a time of life spent among strangers." If this sad commentary carries any truth, it is saddest at death. The final leave-taking most appropriately belongs at home, in the bosoms of those you love.

If you can get it together and assure yourself that these three aspects of pain, tubes, and loneliness will not be yours to bear at the end of your life, then the issue of euthanasia pretty well evaporates. The broad public support of euthanasia results from the sense of disempowerment associated with dying.

A vital way to maintain control over this final passage is the establishment of your wishes with your primary physician, and the reinforcement of a living will or durable power of attorney for health care. I do not want my death to be in someone else's hands, and I intend to make sure that I call the shots. I hope you do, too.

All of us have a right to die, but we also have an equal responsibility to live. Once we have squeezed every drop of good living out of our lives, then the right to die may be asserted. However, insistence on the right to die when there is still abundant living possible diminishes that right.

So live well and fully, *then* die well.

STEP 53. Have Guts

You've got to have guts to grow old. Life courage refers not to a single dramatic act of heroism or death-defying bravado, but to a steady, controlled commitment to facing the tough moments and staying the course. It is a life affirmation. Every life, no matter how seemingly blessed, has multiple episodes of assault and outrageous unfairnesses. If your response to these injustices is to curse the darkness or turn inward to melancholy, then time will not have its chance to play a correcting role. If, however, you are tough enough to face adversity coolly and dispassionately, you can capture the energy of the assaults and turn them to your advantage.

Routinely I see bent, tormented people to whom nature has dealt a cruel hand. I am constantly in awe of the marvelous resilience that many of these people show, and they are great heroes and heroines to me. Just how they got to be that way is obscure to me. Further, they themselves cannot describe where their guts came from. They just have them. Some, when questioned, even assert that the condition that has cursed them has even been a blessing in disguise, as it has shown them how to cope and revealed strengths they didn't otherwise know that they had.

Conversely, I see hordes of patients whose whole lives become unraveled when a minor hurt or loss presumes to come into their lives, and the doctor's office becomes the courtroom for this conflict resolution. Rarely do we physicians cure; always should we comfort. This is a basic premise of medical practice. To comfort is important and appropriate, but this goal should not extend to patronizing. All of us hurt and need comfort at some time or another, yet all of us need courage to see the circumstances in their fullest context and apply our best energies to their solution. Courage by proxy can't work. As a physician, I cannot feel my patient's hurts or comprehend fully the bruises. These hurts and bruises must heal by an innate process. An affirmative approach to life makes the bumps easier to cope with.

As I visualize a human lifespan, it is a bit like a minefield. All over the place, in unexpected places and unexpected times, there are hazards small and large. Of course you need the intelligence not to put your foot down in the wrong place, but more importantly, you need the guts and the courage to venture forth at the onset and to keep going, even while you recognize that danger lurks everywhere.

As you grow old, you should have developed advantages from past experience. You will be accustomed to challenge—how to confront it and steer around it if it is too much, or how to apply its energy to a constructive pursuit. All successful older people demonstrate cool courage and a firm competency that accepts—even seeks—challenge. Without challenge, there can be no flow in life, and not to experience and confront challenges would make life a pretty pallid event. That's why you have to have guts to succeed.

RENEWAL

STEP 54. Recharge Yourself

One of nature's greatest gifts to us is the almost infinite capacity to renew. Rene Dubos delighted in pointing out case after case in which either mankind or a natural force had caused mass devastation to the degree at which any reasonable person would presume that no further life was ever to be possible as a result. But of course a few years later, the renewing process of nature is eagerly at work again. The return of fish to earlier poisoned rivers and lakes, the regrowth of vegetation in scorched Yellowstone, and the healing power of the human body after major injury are all testaments to renewal. I recall well the horror I felt when I viewed the X rays of a dear older friend's leg after a terrible fall. It showed a smashed femur, like a broken piece of pottery. I said to myself that I doubted she would ever walk again. Three months later she was climbing the stairs to the spires of French cathedrals.

The process of renewal almost seems like magic. It reverses apathy, entropy, sullen passivity, grim hopelessness, corrosive melancholy. In retirement and other mid- and late-life disengagements, you are at risk of being relegated to the onlooker bleachers—unproductive, inadequate, and inferior. Renewal is the clear strategy for intercepting the slow drift to premature oblivion.

It is hard for youngsters to grasp the notion of renewability. For them, everything is happening for the first time, and no longitudinal perspective is available when loss occurs. But as someone wisely observed, "It's not how many times you fall down that is important; it's how many times you get up." The advantage of accumulating years is that the reality of renewal is apparent. If you have seen only one springtime eventually following the bleakness of winter, you have no appreciation of renewal. But if you have lived fifty years, you have a serene confidence that spring is soon to come.

Growing older is not the grim slope of decline unsusceptible to renewal. New medical information gives all sorts of evidences that late life is full of opportunities for meaningful activities. In a sense, older people should be more capable of renewal than the younger person with a lesser repertoire of experience from which to draw.

Prospective retirement presents problems: The arenas of income, health, housing, and a purpose in life may all be detrimentally affected. The first three are susceptible to confident coping strategies. The last, finding or keeping a purpose in life, is the area in which the greatest challenge lies. If our late life lacks purpose or necessity, then why renew? Where is the stimulus for regrowth, rebirth, or reaffirmation if life has no purpose? Exploration of the full range of personal potentialities is not something that the self-renewing person leaves to fate. It is something to be pursued systematically to the end of one's days.

Renewability, then, comes down to dependency on just two things—guts and smarts. Smarts means having the competence and accumulated experience on which to depend in asserting the desirability of new action. Guts means having the tenacity and "tough-minded optimism" to see life through. You've heard this before—it applies here as readily as it has previously.

The real prospect of new adventures of body and mind in the decades ahead is one of the real excitements of growing older. We all need more peer examples to show the way—more people in their 90s and beyond who are still renewing. Life and renewability are really synonyms. Life ends when renewal stops.

STEP 55. Stay in Flow

Mihaly Csikszentmihaly's important book *Flow* is full of tips for living a life of optimal experience. It taught me a lot and provides daily evidences of the imperative of staying involved. There is no single way to be involved, no single goal or technique. But it is essential to be involved in something—to be "in flow."

The noted psychologist at the University of Chicago comments on how we are "buffeted by anonymous forces," which make life complicated and uncertain. Only by asserting concerted effort can life have meaning. "The best moments usually occur when a person's body or mind is stretched to its limits by a voluntary effort to accomplish something difficult and worthwhile." Flow exists between anxiety and boredom, between stress and disuse. There is that moment during which we resonate most appropriately and completely with our environment.

Csikszentmihaly's experimental technique reveals that we are in flow when working on a project. My parents taught me that we grow against adversity. When there is no resistance, there is no growth or flow. This is not intuitive. It is not obvious that working would bring more satisfaction than being at idle leisure watching television, but Csikszentmihaly's experiments show a marked distinction between these two activities. "By far the overwhelming proportion of optimal experiences are reported to occur within sequences of activities that are goal directed and bounded by rules."

The implication of these observations to late life cannot be overemphasized. Early in life, your daily activities are largely determined by work or home responsibilities, in which you conform your energies to the obvious tasks in front of you. The principles of *Flow* dictate that you should labor to see that these activities are pursued with enthusiasm and energy, which themselves can become self-fulfilling. Later in life, more time freedom presents itself, and therefore flow activities become more internally generated and directed. If late life dissolves into apathy, boredom, and disengagement, then your flow quotient will suffer badly. Yet if you actively pursue a goal, whether old, new, remodeled, borrowed, or self-generated, then flow presents itself as a lifelong option.

Csikszentmihaly warns us that passivity leads not to a life of gratification but of disillusion. Flow is not a destination, but the journey. It is not so much feeling in control, but of exercising control. It is an active process.

The notion of flow is so inherently congenial to other strategies I've proposed that it reinforces them and is in turn reinforced by them. Daring to be 100 involves effort. It is not a passive gift. It is a treasure to be claimed through the investment of energy, courage, and intelligence. The more resourceful you can remain in all these categories, the greater the proportion of your decades aimed toward 100 you will spend in flow. He or she who dies with the most flow is a success. To be flow-less is a profound tragedy to which too many lives are consigned.

STEP 56. Renew Your Health

Of all your resources, your health is the most precious—more precious than your money, your house, your friends. Without health, everything else becomes a burden. In contrast, with good health almost anything is possible. The best way to save money throughout life is to be healthy. In my family, we have always counted any year in which a doctor (or lawyer) did not have to be consulted as a good year, no matter what else happened.

Of course, health can become expensive when it is lost. There is a corollary myth to the proposition that Social Security will take care of the financial needs of later life, and that is that Medicare takes care of the medical expenses of late life. The latter is no more true than the former. Medicare actually takes care of fewer than half of the medical bills submitted to people over 65. This leaves a large gap, sometimes called Medigap. The entire Medicare payment system should be redesigned. It is philosophically—and threatens to be fiscally—bankrupt. It is an acute phase system attached to a time of life during which chronic problems predominate. It emphasizes efforts to cure, when generally cure is not possible. This is not to say that nothing can be done about late-life medical problems, because there is. But the traditional model doesn't work.

Until a redesign of Medicare takes shape, however, we are left with what we have, which is a mess. Inconsistency, discontinuity, inefficiency, and insufferable complexity are built into the present system. Aging, in the eyes of the major health planners, remains a disease to be cured. Good luck. Instead, they should emphasize function. The major test for late life is whether you can still function, not what diagnosis some physician may have placed on you.

In line with this observation is the unrecognized fact that disability is a much more important health consideration than death. If you are dead, the issues are pretty straightforward. Conversely, disability means you're surviving at a reduced functional level, usually between 20 and 30 percent of maximum vitality, which costs money. It is far better to die from a stroke than to be left paralyzed and speechless for years. Dad used to say to me, "There are lots of worse things in life than dying." Particularly when they are so expensive.

My ideal proposal would be that medical care be delivered to older people largely through the mechanism of a large-scale prepaid plan. For a fixed annual fee, which helps late life planning immeasurably, the system becomes responsible for any and all health-related expenses—disease and otherwise. Such an arrangement would assume the responsibility for health education, preventive maintenance, and crisis care, and finally it would allow people to die at home where they should, not in the indifferent arena of the hospital. A new health professional, cheaper than physicians and nurses, should emerge with competence in the analysis and management of functional decline. There is much positive work to be done, but our present institutions are not well suited to the practical issues at hand.

The best strategy emerges: Live actively and optimistically, and the chances of prolonged frailty are markedly diminished. Then die quickly, at home, with dignity.

STEP 57. Cherish Your World

I grew up in downtown Philadelphia. Trees were scarce in my life. Trolley cars and highrises were my world. The only wild animals I saw were at the zoo. I had no sense of conservation or preservation. My parents didn't understand.

Now the idea of zero environmental impact is a central theme of my life. One of the major contracts that I have made with my planet is that I hope to leave it in better shape than it was when I entered it. This is no slam dunk proposal. I reckon my personal use will have depleted the Earth of several tankers full of fossil fuels. I use my thrice-weekly jogging excursions to keep my neighborhood free of litter. I recycle all I can.

Maybe mine is a feeling of greater responsibility that comes with age, or maybe it is only in our lifetime that we are starting to grapple for the first time with the idea that we are dealing with finite resources. We can't net all the ocean's tuna, cage all the jungle gorillas, or poison all the world's eagles, because there won't be any left. I am secure in the belief that the quality of all our lives will be far richer with the diversity we have inherited than the diminished world our consumption and stupidity threatens to create.

As you age, it is your increasing responsibility to take care of your world, because you have been living in it longer, and therefore it has supplied you with more and been affected more by your usage. You are its patron and shepherd. If you don't care for your world, who will? You are smarter, more informed, and more sensitive to the interconnectedness of things.

Chief Seattle of the Suquamish and Duwamish nations said, "My ancestors said to me, this we know. The earth does not belong to us. We belong to the earth. The voice of my grandmother said to me, teach your children what you have been taught. The earth is our mother. What befalls the earth befalls all the sons and daughters of the earth."

Staying connected with our world has major health implications. If you are indifferent to the health of your Earth, it will deteriorate and adversely affect the life quality of those being born today. Further, insulation from environmental interaction creates a cascade of negative disengagement effects. Just as a leg in a cast shrivels up, so isolating your life from the rest of the life on your planet makes your life wither and makes you a less integrated citizen of the globe.

⌐⌐ STEP 58. Think Travel

Any wish list of things to do during retirement includes travel at the very top. The opportunities that travel offers— adventure, culture, novelty, revisiting, education—have broad appeal to all ages, but retirement offers the crucial advantage of time availability. One of the enlightened provisions of the clinic where I work is the sabbatical. My wife and I have used this time for extended foreign trips to more than fifty countries in Asia, Africa, Europe, and South America, which would not have been possible in the restricted time frames of usual vacations. The experiences we have had have been life shaping for us and for our children. They have provided new understanding, friendships, and perspectives, which otherwise we would lack.

Travel, like other renewal benefits, should be planned. In fact, planning can be a great deal of the fun. Time allows you to take the back roads of the world, the slower carriage, giving you the chance to savor the scenery, since it doesn't flash by so fast. Most midlife travel isn't really travel at all, being more a transfer in time at great speed from one indifferent spot to another. Robert Louis Stevenson wrote, "For my part, I travel not to anywhere, but to go. I travel for travel's sake. The great affair is to move."

Movement and travel for their own sake is a major part of the allure, but learning and involvement in novel experience is implicit in leaving home. Remaining malleable, continuing to grow, is a vital part of aging. Conversely, staying home when opportunity knocks means disengaging from the business of being fully alive. Travel implies continued growth and risk taking. It keeps your brain curious and your dendrites growing.

Retirement travel can have various goals besides geography. Fitness, for example. You may choose an appealing destination because it gives you a chance to climb a peak, take a wonderful hike, or ride a gorgeous river or horse trail. Travel gives you a chance to renew your muscles and bones, as well as your head. Look for travel packages that emphasize sports or other activities.

Older travelers are big business. Many companies cater to older persons, not in a patronizing way, but with designs that can exploit the opportunity, for example, to travel off season. Many colleges sponsor alumni tours, and prestigious organizations such as the Smithsonian offer many ventures, including the opportunity to explore prehistory or attend art or music festivals. Where would you like to go? What would you like to learn? You can choose to share travel with grand-children, explore your genealogical roots, or reacquaint your-self with old friends who also have more time available for adventure. The national park system, with its incredible natu-ral beauties, is an absolute must sometime in life. Travel doesn't have to be to the other side of the world. The next county or valley certainly offers dozens of unexpected trea-sures to explore.

An often unidentified virtue of travel is its ability to foster tolerance. You'll notice similarities more than differences. I find that the older you become, the more patient and under-standing you are of the ways of others. The rough spots, missed connections, and canceled reservations don't seem so critical. The earlier in life such a lesson can be learned, the better, but it is never too late to start.

The major downside to travel is expense. Yes, it must be budgeted for, but senior discounts are almost always avail-able. Numerous package tours offer infinite variety, but often individual travel can be even cheaper. House swaps are often fun and valuable, and there are also opportunities for travel through organizations such as the Peace Corps, which offer the chance not only to see other places and people but also to do something of value for someone else—at no cost.

On whatever level you can achieve it, travel helps life attain a higher meaning.

STEP 59. Think When, Where, and Why Retire

What are you going to do with the rest of your life? If you are planning on dying by the time you are 60 or 70, this question probably doesn't affect you, but what if you plan to live to

100? What are you going to do all those years? Unfortunately, there are no guide books or encyclopedias to provide answers to such a question.

Until recently, the overriding motif for people in their 50s and 60s was that retirement beckoned as a reward for decades at the workbench, a well-earned rest after years of toil. This observation seemed so universal that it seemed it must be right. Its further endorsement by our major institutions—business and government—served to validate its appropriateness. Participation or withdrawal, engagement or disengagement. As the 60s approached, it seemed that it was time to kick back and let someone else carry the load.

But where in nature is there another species in which those in late midlife retire to the treetop, coral ledge, or prairie bunker, tended by the young in reward for services rendered? Retirement, in nature's terms, is an unnatural act. My mentor at the Palo Alto Clinic, Dr. Russel Lee, termed retirement "statutory senility."

A person in his 60s is often in turmoil, repositioning and reapportioning life and future. It can be a time of continued participation or of withdrawal, a time of renewal and engagement or dangerous disengagement. It is clearly a life transition of immense proportion, similar to a marriage, birth, or death. Scholars are split on the health effects of retirement. Many claim no jump up in mortality, while others cite evidence that the retirement years carry many increased risks of physical and emotional decline. Hordes of scientists and philosophers have proclaimed the value of work to human well-being. From the Greeks to Freud, pursuit of a daily endeavor has been viewed as the mainstream of being alive. Loss of this central unifying theme cannot help but be a major juncture in our life trajectory.

Tennessee Ernie Ford sang, "I dig sixteen tons, and what do I get? Another day older and deeper in debt." Good planning does not mean that you must shovel coal or flip burgers or turn screws for 80 years. It does mean that some activity of purpose must prevail—if not coal shoveling or burger flipping or screw turning, then traveling, watching great-grandchildren, or volunteering.

Retirement should be viewed not as a time of rocking chairs, but of trampolines—try out things that have intrigued you, but were never before open to exploration. Think of retirement not as an end but as a beginning, a graduation, a whole set of new opportunities that can enrich and reward. Retirement is an active—not a passive—process. Anticipate it decades in advance, plan for it, and execute it in a well-rehearsed fashion. Of course, this does not imply that it should be rigid in outline. Keep your options open—give new directions a chance. I look forward to retirement in another six years or so, so I can tackle a whole new list of things—joining the Peace Corps, relearning the piano, getting to know my family and friends better. Retirement can and should be the best time of your life—if . . .

ᴶḦ STEP 60. Make Your Last Nest Your Best

I have never heard or read of anyone living all of his or her 100 years in the same home. In our mobile society, we tend to move about every seven or eight years. That would mean on average twelve different homes over a 100-year lifetime.

Like everything else in life, living where you want to live—rather than where you have to live—is paramount. Later in life, the job loses its power as a principal determinant of home site, and new options pop up. Data exist that show that after stopping work, 90 percent of people still live within ten miles of the home occupied before retirement. Further, many of those who have fled south at retirement become disillusioned and return home again. Many of us choose to "age in place."

The most important single issue to be confronted when

DARE to Be 100

approaching the decision of where to live postretirement is the effect any move will have on your overall life quality. Home truly is where the heart is. Several research studies show a strong correlation between longevity and satisfaction with living arrangements. Your lifestyle and the quality of the last phase of your life are primarily dependent on decisions you will make about where you live. Often, late-life home moves can reconsolidate the family, splintered earlier by career demands.

There are a number of lesser variables to consider—cost, climate, safety, tax issues, medical care accessibility, recreation, education, and cultural opportunities. Are pets allowed? If you consider a move to "where the skies are not cloudy all day," visit several times at different seasons to see what summer and winter are like. Subscribe to the local newspaper, and rent before you buy. Develop a sense of how you can become a member of the community, not merely someone on the outside looking in. Life-care communities that provide lifetime medical care are attractive if you crave security and can produce the substantial entrance fee. Other attractive housing models, such as shared living or renting, may be appropriate for you. Renting an extra room of your house to a student might serve both your needs, provided you choose your tenant carefully. I neither encourage nor discourage these varied options—I just present them as choices you might wish to consider.

The least desirable of last homes is an institution where 5 percent or more of inhabitants are 65. Institutional living is hazardous to your health. Institutionalization increases mortality two and one-half fold and represents disengagement with a capital D. Our society must labor earnestly to decrease the need for old age homes.

Stay at home, near people you love and who love you. Keep your home active, living, and involved. Sustain your sense of community, tradition, and continuity. The greenest grass is usually that which you mow yourself.

_⌐_ **STEP 61.** Beware of Retirement Myths

Myth #1. I'll worry about it when the time comes.

Wrong. The abrupt shift in time availability, income, personal relations, and responsibilities that retirement creates bring great discontinuities. Without planning and anticipation, there is often an overwhelming and acute depression, coupled with inaction.

Myth #2. My doctor will take care of my health.

Wrong. Health care is an inside job all the way, and the older you become, the more attention you need to pay. The major issue of late-life health problems is physical dependency. Of the host of things to avoid as you age, dependency is at the top of the list. Let no one else have to wipe your nose or your bottom. Let no one else have to feed you or wheel you. The difference between decades of continued independence or extended dependency is usually a renewed commitment to the pursuit of vigorous health habits. Health is your own job, and retirement often gives you the chance to take even better care of yourself.

Myth #3. The grass is greener down South.

Wrong. Retirement brings with it the unusual opportunity to make a major home move without concern about job requirement. But the loss of continuity with home, family, and community is dangerous. For many, too, the economics that initially appear so inviting become less pleasant when the unexpected happens—such as illness or unanticipated expense. When retirement approaches, you should first explore ways to involve yourself more in your current home and community. The schools, libraries, arts, government need people like you who know the community. Travel, yes, but also stay home.

Myth #4. Of course I will have enough money.

To reach 100? Maybe to reach 75, but have you planned for the long haul? The chances are increasingly strong that you are going to live longer than you had planned. Don't count on Medicare, your pension, or your social security to be enough. The chances are they won't be. Don't be fooled by not investigating. Don't let yourself be surprised, because lack of financial resources is debilitating to morale—it leads to major health problems, which in turn only serve to make matters worse.

Myth #5. Of course I'll have enough to do.

Wrong. Most people at retirement find themselves with too much time on their hands, and TV becomes the easy outlet. If we could capture a small fraction of the wasted hours after retirement, we could start a new world order. Time—not money—is our most precious resource, and its present and future use must be carefully plotted.

The mythology of retirement is not unexpected. After all, we've never really had opportunities like we do now. Let's reappraise and harness the billions of hours of postretirement time to serve the common good. Such an effort will represent a new opportunity of immense proportions.

STEP 62. Afford Retirement

Next year, 2.5 million people will retire. The major attraction and excitement of retirement is the wide range of new options it provides—a new career, part-time employment, volunteer work, or simply the exploration of new uses of leisure. But there is no such thing as free time. Even time costs something.

Regardless of what new path or combination of paths you choose at retirement, it will cost you money.

A magazine advertisement proclaims, "The only thing that is worse than dying is outliving your money." The strategy of bold and intelligent vital living is a certain way of assuring a century of healthy life, but it becomes irrelevant if financial impoverishment looms.

The point, of course, is that your later years, if they are to carry the brightness and promise you anticipate, must have plenty of both health and wealth.

To me, money is just a proxy for energy. I work, and I am paid for my work. I put my money in the bank so I can use it to pay for other people's energy, such as food production or newspapers or musicians or education or gasoline. Over a lifetime, the energies and money have to even out. Fifty years of work at $30,000 a year means $1,500,000 to pay for others' labor and products, spread not just over the years of work, but the entirety of life. This, of course, is where lifelong planning comes in. The checking account needs to show a balance not just at the end of the last month of work, but at the end of the last month of life. If you plan to work all your life, less anticipatory planning is necessary, but if you stop work before the end of your life, saving is beyond option; it is mandatory. We Americans are notable for not being good savers, and in fact we are usually the opposite, debtors. This is not a strategy that can work in retirement. As long as a dependable paycheck is coming in, bills have a way of getting paid, but when the monthly payments stop, bills become less bearable.

Financial planning and savings are the keys to maintaining financial independence as you reach toward 100. Just as you do not want to depend on others to sustain your physical needs as you age, you do not want to depend on children, grandchildren, or anyone else to pay your bills. Being dollar smart in retirement means: (1) planning for your whole life; (2) nonreliance on pensions and social security; (3) considering working for longer than you thought; (4) using principal responsibly; and (5) lobbying for late-life governmental encouragement and incentives.

With proper anticipation, arranging your finances should not be a barrier to reaching 100; instead it should be one of the positive steps you can take to encourage you to reach for that noble goal.

_⌐__ **STEP 63.** Have a Life Money Plan

Having enough money to have a good life is an obvious goal. When confronted by a thief who said, "Your money or your life!" Jack Benny replied, "I'm thinking it over." Retirement and its financial implications must be anticipated. If you wake up on the morning after your retirement, then start to wonder what comes next, you are in deep trouble. I predict your chances of making 100 with such a careless approach to the rest of your life are slim to none.

Having a life money plan carries with it a number of basic elements.

1. Start early. Early savings pay big later dividends. Even small earlier layaways get you into a good habit. Over time, cash equals late-life options.

2. Be steady. Don't look for the early big payout. Delay your gratification to insure late-life financial competence. The chances are that you are going to live a long time, and the steadier you are over the decades, the greater the guarantee of a successful outcome.

3. Stay at risk. As soon as your life money plan turns conservative, you are in danger. Life is inherently perilous, and you must recognize that there is no sure bet.

4. Be flexible. Be willing to transfer from one strategy to an-

other. It is very unlikely that yesterday's plan is still the best for tomorrow. Continue to reassess and rethink. Some expenses—such as housing, education, clothes, and food—usually go down with time. Others—such as travel, entertainment, and health—often go up.

5. Don't be emotional about your program. Be realistic and opportunistic. Don't cling to investments or possessions simply for sentimental reasons. The world changes, and you and your money plan must change with it.

6. Ask for help—but use multiple information sources. Realize that all the experts are there to offer advice more for their benefit than yours. Balance advice and ask for performance records. Beware of commissions.

7. Don't panic about inflation. Sure, your money won't be worth as much next year as this year, but wise investments provide yields that vary with inflation, so the products of your work should not be eroded by inflationary trends. Inflation can vary from 2.5 to 7.5 percent per year, and investments should take this variability into account. Beware of early retirement plans. They are offered to you not for your benefit, but because they will cost the company or government less over time.

8. Be aware not just of your needs but of those around you as well. Share the planning process with your spouse and your children. Ask for their perspectives.

9. Be aware of expenses, as well as income. Both can and will change. What is true of the balance at one time may be totally different at another time. Not spending a dollar is the same as making one. But don't be afraid to spend.

10. If one strategy fails, try another. Don't start with a losing game-plan. Be aware that financial planning implies emotional and physical elements as well. Don't sacrifice one at the cost of another. Life quality is the bottom line.

Planning means staying in charge. It prevents dependency and promotes self-sufficiency. It implies an ongoing involvement in the important domain of active living.

⌐ STEP 64. Be Wealth Fit—Save

Wealth health means having enough not just for today, but for a lot of tomorrows. Wealth fitness means having a balanced approach. This balance is likened by experts to a three-legged stool, the three legs being social security, work income, and savings (including pensions and investments). If you elect not to work, then the other two legs must hold up the stool by themselves. The social security leg is thought by millions of unfortunate people to be enough for wealth health. This is a terrible and dangerous delusion. On average, social security supplies less than 40 percent of late-life income. The modest amount of income available from social security means that the strategy for life savings is paramount to the maintenance of life quality.

A survey conducted by Merrill Lynch revealed that 15 percent of people have no savings plans at all, 39 percent are saving for something other than retirement, and only 35 percent have some retirement savings program, either at work or at home. This figure is only half of what it was a few years ago. We save less than 5 percent of income.

Tens of millions of baby boomers about to turn 50 are at great risk. But, as for all of life's problems, there are solutions: (1) continuing to work; (2) increasing savings; (3) a combination of the two. The prevailing attitude seems to be early, earlier, earliest retirement rather than the reverse. If we dare to be 100, the numbers simply don't add up if you stop working at 62. In 1950 half of the working population still held jobs at 65.

The principal clue to wealth/health success is the length

of the savings period, even more than its industriousness. A dollar saved before 40 years of age equals eight dollars at age 60. Consequently, the longer you can continue to save, the better off you are. Conversely, the longer you work, the more you can save, and it is just in those years between 62 and 70 that the savings can grow dramatically and enhance the value of the savings plan immensely.

The savings aspect of late-life planning is not just bank accounts—by savings I mean home, investments, pensions, and other property. Any wise program tracks all of these assets, then balances and enhances their value. Savings, of course, must include not just your current and future needs, but also those of your dependent family as well. Such savings requires your keeping up to date on current values of each savings category and exploiting opportunities for shifting from one category to another, depending on circumstance.

The other way to save is not to spend. Here is where life quality comes in again. Money is to be used to enhance life quality. If you have the opportunity not to spend without offsetting or improving life quality, then you should take that chance. There are many non-painful strategies to cut down expenses, including selling a second car, discarding excess insurance, and consolidating when possible.

The ultimate value of savings is the number of options it provides. When you have adequate savings, you can be more creative with your work schedule. If your savings are adequate to last until you're 100, then whether to work or not itself becomes an option. Few of us will ever really reach that ideal, however, so the vital advice for us all is to save early and steadily.

The average sum of money Americans have at retirement is $11,000. You'll have to do a lot better than that if you want wealth health.

⌐⌐ **STEP 65.** Keep Working

You are a rare person if, in your mid-60s, you have enough savings to supplement your social security payments and to live carefree to age 100. The three legs of the stool—savings, social security, and work income—will generally require support from all three resources if the best life design is to be preserved.

The desirability of extending the work period of life does not derive only or even predominantly from the financial aspect, although that aspect is not to be undervalued. For most of us, work provides one of our central identities. Retirement provides the opportunity to rethink work. Almost infinite choices exist. Work in the early part of life is mandatory, becoming optional later on. A reworking of the idea of work in your 60s provides you with a treasure load of opportunities, enriched by decades of experiences. You know what you like and what you don't. The financial compulsion of earlier work experience is likely to be less, allowing even more freedom in the choice of a second career.

The first question to ask about your career is whether your current employment situation can accommodate some change; what about job sharing, flexible scheduling, seasonal employment, and other creative opportunities—all of which enlightened corporations and businesses should be inventive enough to explore with you.

Many studies indicate the reliability of older workers, who have lower absentee rates. For the employer, the disadvantage of the older worker generally involves a higher pay category. Certainly your ability to help address this issue, thereby creating opportunities for the upward mobility of younger workers, would be helpful. Or maybe it is time to move on to a new career, a new direction, a new location. Read the want ads, ask colleagues, make new contacts and friends, volunteer to try out some options. Another possibility is starting your own business. Being at risk is part of the idea of continued growth in late life. Or maybe you'll have an opportunity to work from home.

Several Stanford economist friends guessed that if we all really are planning to live to be 100, we need to consider working until we're 80.

Of course, all the central work decisions are best made after you have considered them early in life. I like to create potential work scenarios for the different decades that stretch out ahead.

The image of work as a source of pride—a reason to allow it to control your life—persists. Working yourself to death sometimes doesn't sound like such a bad idea. A regular paycheck is continued evidence of value, currency in fact and meaning. I hope I can be performing labor still worthy of payment as I approach 100. It will mean that my continued existence is necessary to someone else, who also feels my work deserves reward. Continued involvement in active living is the centerpiece of a life fully lived. Continued productivity is a hallmark of successful aging. The clock is not the barrier, and hopefully physical vitality isn't either. Commitment to meaning—in this case to work—is central.

STEP 66. Spend It All

This step is probably the hardest of all to carry out to perfection, requiring both skill and luck. The general principle is to exit life just as you entered it, with nothing. It has never been possible to propose such a step before, because life has been such a crapshoot that all sorts of artificial contingency planning was necessary. Now, however, you can approach your full lifespan with intelligence and confidence.

If you are in the business of planning your whole life in all details, it seems appropriate to consider how much money you want to have in your checking account on the day you die. To me, the clear amount seems to be just what you need: enough to pay your bills and meet your obligations, but no more. The ideal of seeing how large an estate you can accumulate as a marker for a successful life makes no sense to me at all.

The theory goes that if both my wife and I die on or around our 100th birthdays, then our material needs are at an end, and all our accumulated wealth and energies should have been distributed on or about that date. Certainly, emphatically, nothing should be left for the government to come in and plunder. If I care to contribute volitionally to the ongoing financial support of my country before I die, I reserve that right. But the idea that some clown in Washington will lay claim to the product of my life's energies, just because I wasn't smart or careful enough to divest myself of my property (to my family and chosen charities), fills me with horror.

To avoid this fate requires the careful use of principal at the end of life. Reverse mortgages, bequests, and sale or gifts of unnecessary assets should all be deliberately planned. I will never be cash fat, particularly as I die. Save, then use; that is the sound strategy.

I don't pretend that I will ever be smart enough to work out the details of this basic financial planning step, but I commend it to the hordes of financial planners of the world. I am sure that all sorts of tax breaks can accrue if I am smart about using up my estate. I won't need two cars as I die. I won't need even one. I won't need anything, or least that is the grand strategy now. By giving away your assets, you maintain control over your life and your death. I desperately want the satisfaction that what I have spent my lifetime earning is being distributed precisely in the way I want, and the only way to have this confidence is to have an empty checking account when I die. I suggest the same for you.

Some great sage once observed, "You can't take it with you." I have yet to see an exception to this rule, but you can give it away.

⌐ STEP 67. Lobby for Yourself

It is sad but true that the quality of your aging is at least partially in the hands of the government. As you may have noticed, the U.S. government and all lesser state and local variations thereof are not in the business of being responsive and generous to your individual needs as you age. This is not to say that major social programs don't exist that have strong positions bearing on your future, most notably Medicare and Social Security. Unfortunately, however, these "entitlements" create the implication that there is a benign entity out there who is going to take care of you. Wrong! Dangerous and wrong.

Government planning is still the captive of old stereotypes that actually impede reasonable and responsible efforts to live a whole life. Rather than being encouraged, continued involvement is discouraged. Implicit in government tax codes are many incentives to drop out.

Of course, the reverse is true. Income tax rates should decrease with age to encourage active living. The health care crisis would be largely offset if the government offered incentives to remain vital, instead of patronizingly implying, "I'll take care of you."

Government policy encourages dependency. The IRS seems to take perverse delight in changing retirement policy rules, so that sober-minded planning is paralyzed. I do not seek to have the government do more for me or you as we get old. I do seek to have the government enact policies to encourage us to do more for ourselves. Incentives should be provided for healthy behavior. Tax burdens should be imposed on those who thumb their nose at responsible health behavior. The insurance companies have no problem rating teenage male drivers; why can't legislation encourage whole-life living?

As illustrated earlier, it is at the 20 to 30 percent vitality range that health costs accrue. Most of the decay to 30 percent derives from behavioral actions leading to frailty. Frailty costs lots of money and prolongs dying. Active living saves money and shortens dying. We should also consider proposing that no one under the age of 70 be elected to office. In many traditional cultures, a group of people turn to a counsel of elders for advice and wisdom. It makes a lot of sense to me. Older people are destined to be a larger part of the electoral role in the future years. We should use that power wisely and efficiently, not to ask for tax breaks, but for the opportunity to make of our older selves the most we can become. And isn't that the principal task of government in the first place?

STEP 68. Use Leisure

Retirement means the availability of 50 extra hours per week. Multiply 50 hours per week times 35 years, and you have 91,000—a lot of time to spend either in a slow-paced indolence, or embedded in a set of life-affirming growth experiences.

Until recently, abundant leisure time was the exclusive domain either of those who were very rich or very poor. Now, with more generous pensions and social security, so many more have leisure that they feel they can spend the rest of their lives resting up from their decades of hard labor.

You'll notice in these ninety-nine steps to 100, I repeatedly stress the importance of control. Successful living and aging depend ultimately on the maintenance of a sense of control. This is true of new-found leisure as well. If you learn to master your new-found hours, leisure can become a new force in your life. Work, however, is the main source of a sense of control and mastery. When you relinquish it, you are at risk of playing a roleless role. Someone once said, "If what you do is who you are, when you don't you aren't." Leisure can become a stress, a source of inner and outer conflict as the frustration of being viewed as useless breeds aggression and new tension. "Work," said Sir William Osler, "is the master therapy." Leisure is dangerous, unless you use it well.

You need to take control of your leisure, plan it, invest in it, work at it. It is vital that whatever choice you make for involvement must have some meaning for you. Idle immersion or submersion in irrelevant or meaningless activities becomes debilitating and leads to early physical and emotional decay. The greatest potential for meaningful activity is within the family, particularly focused on grandchildren and great-grandchildren. Working mothers increasingly open up the opportunity for retired people to serve an important function for members of younger generations. Outside of family, numerous volunteer opportunities are available to fill for leisure time. Any way you spend it, don't waste leisure.

Disuse atrophy is a well-described medical condition in which parts or all of the body shrivel and deteriorate as a result of disuse. The same is true for leisure activities. If they are allowed to become useless appendages on the tail end of a busy life, then atrophy is sure to follow. An inactive life is entropic and leads to premature aging.

If you are clever, develop an ambitious plan for bountiful use of your leisure—particularly one embedded in extension of family enrichment and growth—and pursue your new life with enthusiasm, then 100 years becomes more and more likely. Good use of leisure time is a major ingredient of a long and worthy life. It helps make sense out of life.

STEP 69. Relearn, Rethink, Reeducate

The greatest treasure you have is not in the bank, but between your ears. That gray corrugated structure, that "computer made of meat" is the seat of your hopes, despair, excitement, loves, creativity, and memories. Your brain changes as you grow older. Time exacts a price on brain power, but this shallow loss is more than compensated for by usage. Brain training provides far greater abilities to a 70-year-old who has used it than a 20-year-old who hasn't.

The brain is elastic. Old brain cells grow new branches when challenged; training can improve late-life learning capacity; and the brain demonstrates an emerging capacity for accumulating wisdom as we age. Older brains can be trained to be much better than they are, as well as much better than they were when they were young.

The later decades not only provide a rich contextual substrate for brain development, but they also provide more of the glorious element, time. You may have heard the saying, "It is what you learn after you know it all that counts." In other words, failures teach, and success is a poor professor. Given the fact that knowledge doubles every ten years, the ability to absorb even a small fraction of this new knowledge empowers our aging. As we age, the relaxation of the hurried urgencies of earlier life avail wonderful opportunities for new learning.

Historian Peter Laslett emphasizes that by only living into our natural lifespan are we able to exploit our true potential. Applying that thought to the power of the mind, if we are dead at 45, our brain hasn't had a real chance to sprout. But if we approach 100, the brain cells can become intimately connected with new and emerging realities.

One of the treasures that we can never have in excess is knowledge. Each new insight, recognition, and experience makes life more valuable. The quality of each day is made better by understanding more. Each of us should be a learning machine.

Not only does knowledge increase the quality of our lives, but there is also ample evidence that it extends the number of our years as well. Smart people live longer. Conversely, when we don't extend our brain power to a sufficient breadth, we fall risk to bad decisions, inactions, and behaviors that are the byproducts of ignorance.

It becomes clear, then, that a lifelong strategy of learning emerges as a potent force for good. Learn everything about something, and something about everything. You'll never be bored if you adopt this approach. You will not only be more valuable to others because of what you know, but to yourself as well, and you'll achieve self-fulfillment and guarantee independence and autonomy—goals all of us cherish.

STEP 70. Sleep Enough

Sleep is the third element of the health triad composed of nutrition, exercise, and rest. Food and activity without adequate rest cannot be sustained without cost. It is true that many of us can go months and even years on four to five hours a night, but the deficit is cumulative and costs us in decreased performance. Sleep deprivation is a national epidemic. Thousands of disasters, small and large, are due to this condition. Beware of "sleep attacks."

Two major synchronizers of your day's wakeful/sleep cycle are light and physical exercise. Both give your brain the cues to say goodnight; however, both of these natural cues have also become distorted by our contemporary existence patterns.

The story becomes even more complicated with older persons. Daily cycles change. Some older people seem to need more sleep, others less, but most tend both to sleep and wake earlier. Their sleep patterns also tend to become more fragmented. Older people spend more time in bed than younger people but may actually sleep less. They have lower levels of arousal, and thus of the good rapid eye movement (REM) sleep. It is difficult to determine if the disturbed sleep of older people results from the process of aging or inactivity. It has been shown that after physical exercise older people experience a substantial decrease in the length of time it takes to fall asleep—and they sleep longer.

There are other ways to alter sleep time: a warm bath two hours before the desired sleep time can often do the trick, as a decrease in body temperature helps promote sleep. Alternately, delay of the evening meal to around 8:00 or 9:00 P.M. can also reset the sleep clock.

The Gallup organization reported that a third of Americans suffer from insomnia, resulting in trouble concentrating, irritability, fatigue, accidents, impaired personal relationships, and difficulty in getting work done during waking hours. This is a huge problem that needs to be addressed, not only by those who identify their insomnia as a problem, but also for most of us as we age. Some things help:

1. Be quiet, dark, and warm.

2. Worry early, not late.

3. Avoid stimulants.

4. Be regular.

5. Have a mate.

6. Be fit.

⌐ STEP 71. Keep in Rhythm

From the lowest creatures on up, we all have living patterns that closely mimic the twenty-four-hour cycle of day and night. There are other time rhythms as well, such as months and years, which are inscribed by events in the sky, but for practical purposes the events controlled by our Earth's rotation are the most important.

Circadian (or daily) rhythms control our lives. Over one hundred separate body functions have been shown to vacillate with cycles related to the time of day; some are fastest or highest in the morning, some in the evening. Some hormones levels can vary fourfold during the course of the day. Body temperature (an important feature, because it controls your metabolism) is highest at midday and lowest at night—not unlike that of the lizard. When the sun comes up and raises its temperature enough to function during the day it is active, but when the sun goes down and its temperature falls, the lizard goes to sleep.

Correspondingly, mental function is higher at midday than at 3:00 A.M. This is due not simply to the sleep deprivation that occurs as the day goes on, but because your brain and body are tightly trained to the twenty-four-hour day/night cycle. Better performances occur at noon during a day following twenty-four hours of sleep deprivation than at 4:00 A.M. following only six hours of sleep loss.

Do you soar with the eagles in the morning or hoot with the owls at night? It's true that many seem to function best after ten o'clock at night—these are the owls. But these people have simply reset their internal clocks. For most, however, the daylight hours are when things get done. Your spirits are brighter, your heart beats faster. There is evidence that the circadian rhythms peak during daytime.

The two dominant forces that reinforce the natural rhythms are light and activity. Some people suffer in varying degrees from the winter blahs, the more severe cases sometimes referred to as seasonal affective disorder. The solution to this condition is more bright light. The common migration south in search of endless summer is a deeply rooted reaction to longer winter nights. Bright illumination, or light therapy, is now recognized as part of the treatment for depression. Similarly, physical exercise is good for your rhythm. When you are physically inactive, your body loses some of its important cues, and your rhythm goes out of sync. This is why, as you age, a regular program of physical activity is essential to good body functioning.

The most obvious distortion of body rhythm occurs with shift work or airplane travel across a number of time zones. It generally takes a shift worker six weeks to readjust to a day-time schedule. Jet lag takes several days to resolve. Careful attention to the resetting of both time and exercise cues leads to easier resolution of the dreary sensations of jet lag and shift change.

Retirement poses challenges to the maintenance of rhythm. Both the retiree and his or her spouse have become used to a rhythm of activity for decades—and all of a sudden this is changed. It is critical to realize that just because you are no longer going to work, the body is still used to a certain level and time of function. If you start to stay in bed later or stay up later at night, your hormones don't recognize this pattern, and you feel out of sorts. On a vacation I have a terrible time "sleeping in," even if I don't have to get up as early as I usually do. If a special occasion means an unusually long evening is coming up, anticipate as best you can, but recognize that it will necessarily take its toll on your rhythm.

Several laboratories are now at work finding out precisely what the chemicals are in your body that control this time pattern. Such information will be interesting, but I doubt that it can ever replace the patterns that have been learned over millions of years of evolution.

Living to be 100 means staying in rhythm. If your life gets too far out of rhythm, the chances are that you won't make it. Learn from experimenting if a walk is best for you in the morning or evening; whether you profit from a midday nap; when your productive work is easiest. Keep your life beat in rhythm.

___

⌐⌐ **STEP 72.** Steps for the Woman

In the perfect world, aging would be sex indifferent, but it isn't. Growing old has markedly different impacts on women and men. Most evident, of course, is the fact that there are so many more women than men. The reason for the difference in lifespan is still not conclusively known, but my deep insight is that it derives from the superior capacity of the female of our species to cope. Many studies have illustrated the strong relationship between ability to cope with adversity and survivability. Men are brittle; women are pliable. The male exists for the moment, the female for the long haul. Nature places a higher value on the female of the species.

Biology, however, does not call the shots at the workplace or in the home, where the notion that "man is king" is still the operative directive. Women's salaries for equal work aren't equal to men's salaries; thereby, pensions and retirement treatments are unequal. Career women also tend to change jobs more frequently than men, further prejudicing their late-life financial well-being. When successful, the triad of marriage, motherhood, and work yields a strong person. The multiple skills necessary to balance these responsibilities are awesome, surpassing any combination we mere males might strive for. The integration of the full woman is a wonder of competence, true beauty, and survivability.

Yet often the full contract is not kept. Too often, we males cop out too early by dying. Widowhood is a major life stress for millions of women, lasting eight years on average. This problem can be largely solved if men simply live longer. But if men exit prematurely, either through death or divorce, the women must survive.

The principal risk of the woman alone in late life is financial. Typically, she has not developed the cash smarts that the man of the house has. He has in most cases made and spent the money. She was on an allowance. Of course, this stereotype is clearly changing, but nonetheless the financial world remains largely male, and in terms of the aging demography, needs to be made much more female friendly.

Any isolation is dangerous, whether biological, psychological, social, or economic. Depression, poor nutrition, lack of physical activity, and fewer social contacts accompany isolation. Living alone is dangerous, as evidenced by the fact that heart attacks are more common in a single person's home. Divorce or widowhood requires the development of new skills. Those who can sustain a support system do well; those who can't fall by the wayside. I have always been intrigued by the unexpected observation that old black women outlive old white women despite their collective health and economic disadvantages. The reason advanced for this observation is that they seem to sustain important family caregiving roles. In other words, they are more *needed*.

The natural nurturing role of women is vital. They find themselves caring not just for themselves, but their parents, children, and sometimes even their grandchildren and extended family. We'd be in a hell of a state without such a female-dominant support system. The self-sufficiency of women is magnificent, not to mention closely aligned with survivability. Most old people—including most centenarians—are women. Older women commit suicide at a rate far lower than that of older males. So in the end, who am I to be telling women how to do anything?

STEP 73. Steps for the Man

There are lots of old men in the world. One was the first ever credentialed by Guinness as having reached 120—Shigecko Isumi of northern Japan—but there are a lot more old women. Men age more quickly and die sooner. Is this due to our nature or our nurture, our genes or our lifestyle?

The answer is still only conjecture. There are clearly major prejudices against men living long. We have higher cholesterol levels, at least earlier in life. This fact alone results in a survival advantage for women. Men indulge in much more self-destructive practices, such as heavy alcohol consumption, smoking, drug use, irresponsible sexual behavior, and fast driving. These behaviors all impact our longevity, but clearly most are, or at least should be, under our direct control.

Job stress, while certainly not uniquely male, is a large contributor to earlier mortality. Yet, as emphasized earlier, it is not the stress itself, but how the individual reacts to it that counts. Despite male bravado and bluster, our ability to stay the course is often defective. Men's rush for immediate gratification, and the emphasis on the moment, are dangerous traits. We understand the time dimension of life much less clearly than women—they nurture time much better than we do.

Grayness, baldness, achiness, sagging, balky prostate—all these so-called age markers afflict men more. Once again, some of these effects are under our control, but the main job of the male life is defined by work and sexuality. How we function in these domains is highly predictive of our life satisfaction. When one or both start to show signs of deterioration or cessation, we perceive that our useful life is threatened. But we must recognize that nothing in nature ever stays the same. Change is inevitable. Nevertheless, we can rationally confront job and sexual change. No, we will not be the same man at 80 as we were at 20, but there can be offsetting gains. Job alternatives are abundant, and I am very hopeful that science will soon give us better coping strategies for sexual change as well. As we harness these strategies, we men will have a better chance of sharing 100 with our mates and families.

EXERCISE

Ten reasons not to exercise:

1. I don't have time.

2. I can't exercise because I'm out of shape.

3. If I exercise, any time that I will live longer I will have spent exercising, and therefore I will have wasted it.

4. I don't enjoy it.

5. If I exercise, I might not have enough energy left over for sex.

6. The TV at the gym is always tuned to something I don't want to watch.

7. It will ruin my eye makeup, or my hair might get messed up.

8. My uterus might fall out.

9. If I exercise, I'll get hungrier, so I'll get fatter.

10. Sweating makes my eyes hurt.

Now, twenty-six ways to counteract these.

STEP 74. Take the First Step

The first step is the hardest and most important. But once you start, you have got to keep going. Good intentions remain only good intentions until you follow them with action.

Different people obviously have different reasons to start to exercise, and even more reasons not to exercise. Very few, if any, are legitimate, particularly age. The thought "I'm too old to exercise" should be translated into "I'm too old *not* to exercise."

The first step is to establish incremental efforts. Don't try to run a mile or swim the width of the lake the first week. Walk around the block or swim a few yards in the pool first. Develop your confidence and your new self-identity as an active person. There is no need whatsoever to do it all at once. See what works and what doesn't. Alone or with someone else? In the morning or the evening?

The second step is to seek peer examples. Find other people like you who are active. Find out how they started and what keeps them going. Find out all about them—their schedules, their nutrition and sleep habits, and what problems they have had along the way. There is not a fit person in the world who hasn't experienced periods of doubt along the way. Find out from others like yourself what works for them, and then adapt this strategy for yourself.

The third step to sustaining fitness is to collect information about the active lifestyle. There is an ever-growing data base that makes a fit life more appealing. The more you learn, the more you will identify how this critical commitment will benefit every one of the rest of your days. Don't just rely on your physician, although he or she should be an active ally in your effort. Hopefully your family will participate as well, and as all of you learn and relearn the value of staying fit, the hard times will seem easier.

The fourth step is the diminishment of the cues of failure, such as stiffness, blisters, or fatigue. Every time you stretch yourself and your competence, your mind and body must also stretch to include your new ability. There will, of course, be growing pains. I am always aching on the mornings when I extend my jogging miles in anticipation of running a marathon. But the aches are minor, disappear after a few minutes, and are actually an integral part of becoming better conditioned.

With these first four steps, you will be able not only to start but to sustain an exercise program. I often recommend Ken Cooper's famous book *Aerobics* to my patients, as it provides strategies on how to build up and sustain such a program. The more you do, the more confident you will become, and the more self-esteem you will acquire. The result will be your sense of mastery not only over the exercise but over yourself as well.

⌐⌐⌐ **STEP 75.** Know How Hard, How Long, How Often to Exercise

The tremendous value that physical exercise provides to your body is established beyond any reasonable doubt. Dr. Bob Butler said, "If there were a drug that provided all the benefits that exercise does, the whole world would be taking it." Of course, there is no such drug; the value of exercise must come from an activity program of your own devising and accomplishment. You cannot delegate exercise, and you can't get something for nothing.

The overall basic truth is clear. What remains are the details. How hard must you exercise, how long, and how often? Is what counts the total amount of exercise—regardless of the duration or single bursts of activity? Further, a certain duration, frequency, and intensity of exercise may be best for one condition—lower blood pressure, for example—whereas another combination of exercises may be best for weight control. Also important to note is whether the exercise prescription is for prevention or treatment of a condition. All the details and variables must still be worked out.

The prescription of a half hour per session, three times per week, at an intensity hard enough to make your heart pound, make you sweat, and induce only minimal difficulty while carrying out a conversation still remains the departure point for the health value of exercise. Spurts of exercise that are more frequent, less vigorous, and shorter, or less frequent, more vigorous, and longer are all valuable, as long as they are not too strenuous. The phrase "No pain, no gain" has been retranslated to "less pain, more gain." The more intense, frequent, and longer the workouts, the more chance there is for injury and decreased immune response. The less active, less frequent, and shorter, the less benefit you'll derive. As with most things, moderation seems best.

Anthropologists tell us that the hunter-gatherer took care

of his or her food needs by hunting three times per week for a half hour or so each time. This schedule bears a striking similarity to the best prescription for contemporary exercise. It is likely that what we did for nearly four million years, until civilization changed our lifestyle, comes down to us as a basic survival strategy. What our forebears did to survive likely represents what we need to do to survive, too. Make your exercise strong enough, but not too strong; often enough, but not too often; long enough, but not too long. You'll find your pace, but only if you start and sustain.

STEP 76. Realize It's Never Too Late

"I wish I had started sooner."

Nature has an almost infinite capacity for renewal. An old tree still grows branches; an old ram still grows horns. Nature preserves growth capacity, as long as favorable conditions are maintained, including use. When you stop using yourself, you decay rapidly.

In the ideal world, we would all be wonderfully fit and would have exercised over all our lives. However, this is rarely the case. Often there are accidents or other episodes that get in the way of remaining active. More of us seem simply become bored and disinterested and develop an inertia that makes us fall off the fitness bandwagon and join the ranks of the couch potatoes.

The best example of the resilience of the body is the widely cited work of Maria Fiatarone in Boston. Maria selected the frailest among us—90-year-old nursing home residents—and measured their muscle size and strength. If there were any group for whom you might presume it's too late to start exercising, it would be these people. But you'd be wrong. Just a few weeks of a strengthening program resulted in bigger, stronger muscles and fewer falls. More than any other study, Maria's work refutes the idea that it is ever too late to start becoming fit. It contradicts the age prejudice that too many of my physician colleagues assert when they make negative treatment judgments about a patient, simply because of birth date.

Fitness for a young person is an option. Fitness for older people is an imperative. As I have already stated, a fit person of 70 is similar to an unfit person of 30.

That it is still possible for older people to become fit should come as no surprise. It is nature's way of guaranteeing survival. Older brains, like older muscles and hearts, respond vitally to use.

When my older patients tell me of their inactivity and offer age as an excuse, I immediately counter with stories of individuals such as Ivor Welsh and Paul Spangler, who didn't run until late in their lives and were able to run full marathons of twenty-six miles into their 90s. It is not age but desire that determines the boundaries of physical activity. The accomplishments of older athletes are amazing and only getting better. Some performances of athletes in their 70s and beyond are strong enough to have won them Olympic medals fifty years ago. I anticipate the day, not far away, when centenarians will be boasting performances that once were held to be those of only highly gifted athletes.

When an old clock stops, it is usually not because it is broken or is worn out, but because it needs to be wound. You are no different from a clock. Keep yourself wound up.

⌐ **STEP 77.** Make Time for Exercise

It is easy to advise when not to exercise—after a big meal, in the extreme heat or cold, first thing in the morning, without a warmup or proper conditioning. These circumstances are just plain dangerous. One experiment took a group of supposedly healthy men and performed an electrocardiogram on them following fifteen seconds of sudden hard exercise. Seventy percent displayed an obvious heart abnormality. When the same men were allowed a warm-up before the strenuous workout, however, virtually all showed a normal response. Clearly the *when* to exercise is significant.

We are so busy riding that we don't have time to walk anymore. The excuse that there is no time for exercise is not acceptable. An adequate physical fitness program requires no more than 3 hours out of 168, only 2 percent of the week's time. Three hours of life can be gained for every hour spent exercising—a good bargain, no?

When should you exercise? It is interesting to note that most track and field and weight-lifting records have been set in the afternoon. By afternoon, muscles have had a chance to loosen up and become nourished by an overnight rest. Weight lifters clearly indicate that their ability to pump iron is better after their muscles have been warmed up.

It is also not coincidental that most heart attacks seem to occur early in the morning, before the body has had a chance to wake up. At that hour, the heart is faced with the task of kicking into activity before it is ready. It becomes stressed, and damage occurs. Any sensible athlete's workout will include a warm-up period first. This advice is most important for the weekend warrior, who recalls days from decades past when he or she was fit and performing at high levels. Foolishly, this individual tries to pick up where he or she left off, and a high-danger activity results.

The timing of exercise is not so crucial. What is crucial is that it is done regularly—not episodically, in extreme cold or heat, or in an initial burst.

The timing of exercise affects the timing of eating, and vice versa. You shouldn't eat before you exercise. Your mother taught you that years ago. You *should* eat afterwards. This is when the muscles are particularly subject to energy replenishment. Eating makes the blood go to the stomach and deprives the muscles that are being exerted. Our hunter-gatherer ancestors hunted and exercised when they were hungry, not when they were full. We should follow their example.

Make time for exercise. Your life—and its quality—depends upon it.

STEP 78. When Tired, Exercise

"Doctor, I'm so tired." I would guess that this is the most common complaint I hear in my office. Millions of dollars are spent in the effort to stamp out fatigue. Usually the cause is obscure, the possibilities many.

After failing to find a medical reason for the fatigue, I inquire about life habits. How are you sleeping? How's your diet? Are you getting enough exercise? I would venture a guess that in my practice it is in this series of questions that the basic answer to the problem of fatigue arises. Remember that most of my patients are old, and fatigue is a very common complaint. Just a simple inventory of rest, food, and activity patterns often reveals major problems. These errors in living often have a social root. No one to cook or shop with, fear of being, walking, eating alone. My hunch is that millions of Americans do not venture out simply because there is no one there to walk with. My further guess is that if we had some basic social institutions that would encourage, assist, or in any way facilitate an expanded opportunity for older people to walk, this congenial step would do more good for millions of older people's fatigue than any other action. Frequently an older person arrives in my office in a wheelchair, and I ask why he is in the chair. "Why, Doc, I'm eighty-five" is the common response. I react, "What's eighty-five got to do with it? I know people in their nineties who are still running marathons!" Yet the perception remains that being old somehow provides an excuse for inactivity—and almost certainly fatigue follows.

Another cause for fatigue may be depression. Any discussion of depression mentions chronic overwhelming fatigue as one of the most common symptoms. Inactivity breeds depression, and depression breeds inactivity in an endless cycle. Earlier I mentioned the central role of exercise as a therapy for depression. It breaks the vicious cycle.

Exercise is its own reward over and over. But its role as a fatigue fighter is supreme. Rather than lying down when you feel tired, take a walk, go for a bike ride, take a swim. I promise you you'll feel better.

Obviously, exercise isn't the answer to all complaints of fatigue, but it comes closer than anything else I know. Out-of-shape America gets tired too easily. It needs a transfusion of energy. This prescription starts at home. It is cheap, safe, and almost universally effective. Give it a try.

STEP 79. Don't Fear Exercise

It used to bother me when my patients, knowing of my commitment to exercise, would come into my office and throw down a newspaper clipping relating the death of someone who died while jogging. Such rare events are newsworthy, as they seem to contradict the supposed life-extending benefits of exercise. But there are no stories about people who suffer a fatal heart attack while sleeping or eating, and we continue to practice these behaviors anyway. Nevertheless, it bothered me that implications might be drawn from the reports of "jogging deaths." It is hard enough to get the couch potato to consider exercise without his worrying that he might die as a result. However, I now take the reverse strategy in responding to this challenge. I assert that "I hope I, too, die while jogging, or making love, or climbing a tree. I don't want to die in bed." I hope my boldness rubs off on others.

Ever since Pheidippides collapsed and died after running from Marathon to Athens to report the defeat of Sparta, strenuous exertion has worn a caution label. "Careful. Physical exercise may be dangerous to your health" is a commonly heard refrain, and several recent deaths of star athletes during games have accelerated the concern. Dr. Paul Thompson at the University of Pittsburgh concluded that there is one death per 396,000 hours of exercise. This is one for every fifty years of heavy work. Said in another way, there is one death per 18,000 exercisers per year. These numbers are very small. Every year many runners run marathons, even though they have had prior heart attacks, heart surgery, and even heart transplants. Exercise is good for hearts.

Life is always an uncertain affair, but there are preventive steps you can take to guard against bad exercise-related events. The best defense is smarts. If you have unusual shortness of breath, chest pain, heart skips, or if risk factors such as cigarette smoking, high blood cholesterol, bad family history, heart medicines, or high blood pressure play a part in your life, you better get a doctor's clearance before exercising. This does not mean, however, that most people need a full-scale checkup before embarking on an exercise program. With common sense as a guide, most people can exercise without problem, even past age 70.

A slow, steady, regular exercise program is one of the safest and surest ways of daring to be 100. Like other dares, the better you are informed about the risks and the way you can offset them, the better off you are. Take the commonsense approach and don't exercise when it is too cold or hot, when you are sick, too soon after eating, or in a hostile place. As always, there are negatives to anything that is valuable. This is why I hope I do die while doing something active.

STEP 80. Don't Say, "I Don't Want to Lose It, But It Hurts Too Much to Use It"

Injuries are a major deterrent to exercise. Knowing when a pain is a command to slow down or stop is an important part of any active life. The human body is a healing machine, and even a badly smashed bone is strong again in six weeks if it is allowed to heal.

Every person without exception who lives an active life will have injuries. It is part of the process, and the body's capacity to repair itself is virtually limitless. But—and this is an important but—there are rules to follow. If a fellow comes to my office and tells me he turned his ankle three months ago and it still hurts now, I ask immediately what he has been doing during this time. If he sheepishly confesses that he is jumping rope three times a day, I explain that obviously the body can't heal itself if he insists on abusing it.

The other important aspect to consider, however, is the mechanical soundness of your body. If you have a joint that is off angle, bowed legs, or crooked knees, continued use will apply inappropriate and excessive forces on the tissue, and any use will encourage reinjury. But if the joint is stable, then use is good for it. Swelling, redness, and prolonged tenderness are the three signs that you should back off and allow healing time.

Joints are meant to be used. Obviously each joint has a maximum amount of pressure it can withstand. Overload—pushing a joint past its maximum—causes problems, but underload does, too. Each of us is so wonderfully made that the range between too much and too little is very wide.

Some muscle soreness and stiffness is natural after exercise, particularly if it is more than usual exertion. Sometimes the soreness may take two or three days to develop, a process called DOMS (delayed onset muscle soreness) that's due to spasms, stretches, and even little tears in the muscle tendons. You can avoid DOMS with a gentle warm-up, and the more fit you become, the less DOMS you will experience.

What about the person with arthritis? It used to be said that the treatment for a sore joint was permanent rest. No more. Now we know that any joint that has arthritis in it must enjoy sustained exercise to maintain its function. Of course, this doesn't mean stressing a joint that is actively inflamed; such inflammation must be allowed to heal. But once healing is complete, the ligaments, tendons, and muscle fibers that hold the joint in its best alignment must continue to be used. A recent report published in the *Annals of Internal Medicine* showed that an eight-week walking, stretching, and strengthening program involving a hundred people with arthritic knees not only increased their ability by 30 percent, but lowered pain 27 percent as well.

Ice and anti-inflammatory medicines help shorten the recovery from pain. But the body is wise. Listen to it, and you will sense when your joints are meant to move. Not moving is unnatural. You pay a price when you don't move. Don't be afraid of soreness—it can be your badge of involvement. Rest and then move on.

STEP 81. Watch Your Fuel Gauge

A car gets so many miles to the gallon. Any engine when it is turned on needs a certain amount of power to run. When it is not turned on, it doesn't need any fuel. You are the same. If you sit in idle you need very little fuel, about one calorie per minute just to keep your engine in neutral. When you put your body in gear, however, it needs a lot more energy. A muscle at rest needs only a smidge of food fuel to stay alive, but when it is used, its energy demand may go up seventyfold. Some very active people may need 6,000 calories per day just to maintain their body weight. Inactive people, on the other hand, may need only 1,000. So the range of food calories your body needs may be quite broad, depending on how you run your machine.

The standard unit of calorie need is 100 calories per mile. Running a mile also requires 100 calories, only it is burned faster. So clearly the intensity of the exercise affects how rapidly the food is burned. Light exercise is generally thought to be activity that requires about three times the basic caloric need (called 1 met, for metabolic equivalent). Really heavy work may require ten times the basic (10 mets); housework is generally 2 to 3 mets in intensity. Although it is impossible, without being in a laboratory, to know precisely how many calories you are burning while doing anything, your pulse rate is a rough guide. The harder you are working, the more oxygen and calories you will burn, and the faster your heart will beat.

A pound of body fat contains 3,500 calories, so if one of the purposes for your exercise is to get rid of excess pounds, you can figure out how long it will take at what workload. One pound of fat equals thirty-five miles of walking or running, seven hours of gardening, or eight hours of golf. This may seem like a harsh bargain, but it's not so bad as it sounds. Exercise helps burn calories and fat, not just for the time spent doing it, but especially afterward. The afterburn of exercise is significant. For several hours after exercise, the body is still burning, unlike the time during or following TV watching.

The way to relate calories to exercise is to put it into a time perspective. If you jog, swim, bike, jump rope, play volleyball, or climb stairs for one hour three times a week for eight weeks, you will lose five pounds. Carry these calculations out to a year, and you can see what a difference an exercise commitment makes to your calorie count.

Keep your machinery running hard enough, often enough, and long enough, and the fuel balance pretty much takes care of itself. If you insist on being inactive, however, then you will be part of the fat, unfit America that costs everyone too much in health-care expenses, not to mention doesn't have a chance of reaching 100.

⌐⌐ **STEP 82.** Learn with What and When to Fuel the Exercise

The *why* of exercise is easy. The *what* and *where* are less clear. How to fuel the physical activity requires insight. The adage "Never eat right before you go swimming" contains some truth. After eating, quite a lot of blood is diverted to the stomach and intestinal tract to help in digestion. Several studies have shown that eating half an hour before some exercise actually cuts down on performance. If you start to exercise then, routing blood to the muscles, you set up a competition. Ideally you should exercise three hours after having eaten, thus allowing all the food to be out of the stomach. High-fat foods take longer to empty out, so the pre-exercise meal should consist mostly of carbohydrates.

The main fuel used in exercise is not the meal eaten immediately before, but the stored-up glycogen (carbohydrate) and body fat that is released from the body stores during any prolonged exercise. Some exercise trainers recommend carbo-loading before an endurance event such as a marathon, which is why the prerace pasta dinner has become a ritual.

One important point to make concerning food and exercise is never to try some new formula for the first time on the day of an event. Any experimenting with food or fluid mixture should be done at a time when you are not expecting a special performance. The basic truth is that it is the well-balanced nutritional format that best serves exercise needs. The more you exercise, the more food you need. And the more food you need, the greater the likelihood that your diet will include enough of all the basic requirements. Therefore, a pretty sure way of insuring an adequate diet is to exercise. This advice may seem the reverse of what it ought to be, but it works, particularly in our sedentary world.

Some prohibitions are clear. Alcohol and exercise don't mix at any age, but particularly as you grow older; alcohol causes shifts in metabolism, impeding performance. Too much caffeine tends to be dehydrating. TV addiction is bad, really bad, as it inhibits exercise, but it represents a double negative, because the hours of inactivity are often accompanied by the ingestion of junk food, which compounds the activity by sludging up the system.

As you commit to a lifelong program of exercise, knowing the *whats, wheres,* and *whys* of food is helpful. Ensure that your energy will not sputter and falter, that it will carry you the whole journey. Over a lifetime of 100 years, your body manages 70 million calories, a huge number, which speaks strongly for how efficient your machine is—if you don't junk it up.

STEP 83. Keep Your Oxygen Tanks Full

Think for a minute of what your body does. It eats, it drinks, it breathes, it thinks, it makes love. But you don't have to think to survive (many people go lifetimes without ever having had a meaningful thought). You don't have to make love to live (though it wouldn't be nearly so much fun). You can live weeks without eating and days without drinking, but you can only go a few fragile minutes without breathing. Like a candle under glass, you extinguish very promptly without oxygen. Your brain can stand about four minutes without the circulation that brings its oxygen supply to it.

Your ability to absorb oxygen from the atmosphere and move it through the channels of your body—trachea, bronchi, lungs, arteries, capillaries—to the cells where it is used to burn food fuel is absolutely dependent on your physical fitness. A fit person of 70 has the same capacity to move oxygen into the body as an unfit person forty years younger. Fitness is therefore a forty-year age offset when it comes to oxygen usage.

This is about as good a measure of body vitality as I can imagine. Without a good system of oxygen delivery, it is still possible to live (for example, think of the person who suffers from advanced emphysema), but with a lifetime tied to the oxygen tank, the quality of life is vastly diminished.

Oxygen-carrying capacity goes down as the result of age change, but it does so only at a very slow pace. If you are fit, your oxygen supply should carry you easily to 100. However, if you are unfit, you lose your oxygen-transporting capacity about four times as fast as you would if you were fit, so by the time you are 70, you are short of breath, and even a little effort makes you puff. Such conditions accelerate—the less you can do, the less you will do—until you become armchair bound, all because you have lost your oxygen fitness.

Why does physical fitness help you carry oxygen? Mainly because virtually every step in the delivery process is kept at optimum functioning level through usage. The lungs, heart, arteries, head, and metabolic machinery of the cells are all kept oiled and efficient by continued use.

Many people are enthusiastic about meditation and relaxation as keys to a long life. I am, too, but they are not enough. These techniques help even out the frenzy bumps that life presents, but they don't increase your oxygen-carrying capacity. I like to think that my jogging exercise program gives me both. Not only does it provide meditative periods of contemplation and peace, but it also pumps up my ability to move oxygen.

If you hope to be 100 and vigorous, you need to burn oxygen. It provides your flame and brightness, and without it your embers dim. Fan the flames. Exercise.

STEP 84. Make Exercise Your Circulation's Best Friend

Heart disease is the biggest killer, but it's slightly misnamed. The real culprit is artery disease. Those thousands of pipes that connect your heart to everything else carry the food and oxygen for life. When they are clogged with clot or cholesterol, they fail in their function, and damage ensues.

A program of lifelong physical exercise is the single most important protection against stopped-up pipes and heart trouble. Exercise confers major advantages on virtually every step in the process that leads to circulatory collapse. Once a heart attack or stroke has occurred, a cure is not only unlikely, but impossible. The doctors struggle to preserve what is left, but when the damage is already done, permanent injury results.

One reason that the recognition of exercise's preventive force in heart and artery trouble has taken so long to be appreciated is the numbers of reports that indicated the relatively short life expectancy of college athletes. If exercise were good for you, how come these stars failed to live long lives? The answer now is very simple. Merely because an individual was fit in his or her 20s means little if the level of fitness isn't sustained into the 60s and beyond. To provide value, physical exercise must be a lifelong habit.

The benefits exercise brings to the fight against heart disease are huge. All of the factors that contribute to heart attacks because of blocked arteries can be addressed by exercise. Not only does exercise help lower the total blood cholesterol levels, but it alters the types of cholesterol as well. Exercise also helps lower the blood pressure. As you no doubt know, people with higher blood pressure run higher risks of heart disease. When you exercise, your arteries dilate, and thus the blood has a larger volume within which to be distributed, and in turn blood pressure falls.

Want more evidence? Exercise helps smokers quit. Cigarette smoking is a strong predictor of early heart problems. Almost no one who is physically active smokes. Rather than my trying to convince my heart disease patients to stop smoking, I instead encourage them to start to exercise. It is easier to engage in positive behavior than to stop negative behavior.

More? Exercise cuts down the clottability of blood, so it is less likely that a block will occur in a crucial artery. There are many medical efforts to thin the blood of people with heart disease. Exercise does it naturally. Finally, exercise enlarges the arteries. Larger arteries can tolerate more cholesterol sludge passing through.

All of these—and more—provide ample incentive to be fit. Heart surgeons and undertakers probably won't like it, but as you become better conditioned, your arteries and your heart will thank you for preserving their ability to keep the juices flowing.

STEP 85. Be Strong

If you are planning a long trip, you want to be sure that whatever kind of conveyance you are planning to use for your trip is sturdy enough to carry you the whole way and not leave you broken down before the trip is over. But what if your trip is 100 years long and your vehicle is your body? Will it last you your full lifespan?

There are many, many reports of the large number of people who are 80 years old and can no longer climb a flight of stairs, lift ten pounds, or even get out of a chair. Some can't dress, feed themselves, or get to the toilet alone. A great many are frail. The large number of frail older people are not frail because they are old—or even because they are sick. They are frail because they stopped moving. They have abandoned the energetic part of their lives and become dependent on machines and other people to do their moving for them.

Each of the 430 voluntary muscles of your body is there to be used—this means both contracted and stretched. If a muscle isn't used it shrinks. When sidetracked from use, muscles lose their strength at 1 percent per day. Obviously, decades of indolence lead to muscles that are mushy and ineffective.

Very few of us have occupations that ensure lifelong muscle strength. The truth is that virtually no sport conveys the ideal strengthening program for your whole body, and therefore you need a muscle program as a life strategy—much like the way you bathe or brush your teeth.

Strengthening does not require fancy equipment. A detergent bottle filled with sand, cans of food, inner tubes, or socks filled with pebbles serve as effective exercise aids. A simple broom handle is an excellent tool to use with an exercise partner in such ways in which two people can benefit from the exercise at the same time. Music is a common and pleasant accompaniment to the activity.

The basic principles of the program are few:

1. Start slow, go slow. Don't push it, but keep it up.

2. Try to have a schedule that will provide two or three workouts each week.

3. Each muscle should be put through its full range of motion. Being musclebound simply means that a muscle isn't stretched through its entire arch during the strengthening process.

4. The exercise program should be designed so that each movement is repeated approximately eight times in a sequence.

5. Use standing, sitting, and lying as starting postures for the exercises, because each one provides a chance to use different muscle groups.

6. Lift weights (isotonic strengthening) instead of pushing against a fixed object (isometric strengthening).

7. Increase the amount of weight you use gradually. Never overextend. Your aim is not to be the strongest person in the world—not even the strongest you—only a strong-enough you.

8. Inhale before you lift, exhale as you lift. Never hold your breath. Each movement takes around fifteen seconds; seven seconds up, seven seconds down.

9. If you are very sore after a workout, you have overdone. Back off and resume at a lower workload.

Being strong confers all types of advantages. You improve your circulation, spirits, balance, and resistance. An added bonus is that you can do more the next time. Remember, you can't move mountains if you can't move yourself.

STEP 86. Stay Loose

Stretching probably gets even more important as you age because stiffness and loss of elasticity are part of the aging process. For evidence of this loss, pinch the skin on the back of your hand and watch how long it takes to regain its form. The same process happens to muscles, tendons, and ligaments. Cross-linkage occurs, which means that molecules get locked together, like ice crystals. To slide them takes more effort.

Your back is probably the most sensitive target for stiffness. Back pain is probably due both to muscle weakness and stiffness. The same goes for the neck. The answer to both the back and neck problems is stretching. Be sure you put your muscles through their full range of exertion at least twice each week and in a set of repetitions that ideally accompany the flexing and strengthening exercises.

In stretching, it is important not to bounce the stretch or overstretch, because that is a sure way to be injured. Overpulling or overstretching simply extends muscle fibers more than they are intended to stretch. As an example, think about whiplash to the neck, in which the neck is suddenly whipped through an unnatural arc, resulting in a hyperextension injury. Whenever a muscle or tendon is overstretched and injured, the treatment should be similar to that for an overflex-ion injury—rest, ice, and anti-inflammatory medicine. Virtually all overextensions heal by themselves.

Again, the more you stretch, the easier it becomes and the less prone to injury you will become. All top athletes have learned to stretch because they realize that their downtime due to injury will be reduced if their tissues are supple.

And don't forget that smiling, too, is a wonderful stretching exercise. The more you smile, the better your face will feel—and the better other people will feel, too.

Don't get tied up in knots; instead, stay loose. It is much better to be a loose 100 than a tight one. When you die, you get stiff pretty quick. No sense in speeding it up.

STEP 87. Stay Balanced

Statistics reveal that one in every three persons over the age of 75 suffers from at least one major fall each year. The frailer you become, the more you fall. Accidents are the seventh leading cause of death in persons over 75, with falls accounting for the majority. Falls contribute to insecurity, so when an older person falls, he or she is less likely to remain active, and the stage is set for increased inactivity, fragility, and further falls. Arthritis, circulatory troubles, and poor vision contribute further to instability and potentially dangerous tumbles.

When bones are fragile, even a slight fall may result in a fracture. There are 250,000 hip fractures per year in America, 20 percent of which lead to a fatality, either directly or indirectly.

So the issue of decreased balance as you age is a major one, one to be addressed before the fact rather than after. Those in midlife should include balance exercises in their repertoire of fitness workouts. A study by Leslie Wolfson at the University of Connecticut found that three months of training a group of persons over 70 years of age improved their balance 100 percent. Dr. Mary Tinetti emphasizes that muscle strengthening, particularly around the ankle, is important for protection against falls. Good shoes are also important.

Increasingly, I advise my patients to maintain their balance through practice. Be a flamingo. One simple exercise consists of standing on one leg for half a minute, then the other—four or five minutes a day. This exercise is made more challenging by closing your eyes. The trick is to start out doing the one-leg stands while hanging onto the back of a chair (with both hands if necessary), then gradually progressing to one hand and eventually one finger—before performing the exercise with no aid at all. Tai-chi, a Chinese program of balance and meditation, is another wonderful alternative for strengthening balance and confidence.

Aerobic fitness, strength, and flexibility are all necessary in their own right, but without balance, the other elements are insufficient. Our gyroscopes need to be kept fine tuned. The more you use balance machinery—with its various component parts—the steadier you will become. And the more fit you are (in the broadest sense), the more secure your stability will be as you move through your later years.

_⌐_ **STEP 88.** Stand Straight

Be an exclamation point, not a comma. Stay in line. Don't sag. Stand tall. Keep your eyes on the horizon, not on the ground just in front of you.

Some of the bad news about aging derives simply from the way many older people look. They look bent and spent. Their posture seems to tell the story of their lives, as drooping slowly to the grave. Of course, almost all of this is preventable, and much of it is reversible. The dowager hump comes from decades of conceding to gravity—and just plain laziness. You have to work to have good posture.

Good posture depends on having a good girder structure. When the girders are straight, they hold the body in its best design, and all your organs have their proper settings. They belong where they are. If through bad posture you end up relocating them, however, they won't work as well. Consider your lungs. Early in life, they have a fine chamber—the chest—to ventilate within. The full excursion of the diaphragm allows you to move gallons of fresh air in and out. But try taking a deep breath when you are bent over at the waist. The bellows of your chest simply can't work when you are stooped. Further, bad posture puts tensions on the fibers of your diaphragm, which in aging can weaken enough to lead to a hiatal hernia of the stomach up into the chest, which complicates breathing further and often creates digestive problems. Living in a bent position compromises good digestion. Try curling up right after a big meal. It doesn't feel good.

But the biggest problem the late-life sags create is on the spine. The spine is the centerpiece of posture and is most affected by it. With its many intersecting joints of the vertebrae, its proper alignment is crucial. This alignment is guaranteed by the pulls and counterpulls of the back and belly muscles. When these steadying forces are malaligned, either by poor habit or muscle weakness, the spinal joints start to rub, irritating each other and producing arthritis. Everyone should do exercises regularly to ensure that the precious joints of their spines are well maintained in their proper alignment. The arthritic process is made worse, too, by the common bad actor, obesity. The added burden of weight upon the spine further encourages bad posture habits by laying extra force on the vertebral joints. The process then becomes self-accelerating. The more the spine tips, the more it tends to tip. It is sturdiest when it is straight.

As you age, posture becomes more important. It is an emblem. A straight back in a 90-year-old is a credential of a life actively lived. It seems to convey an optimistic attitude. It reduces wrinkles. Every physician is aware of the condition know as contractures, in which a part of the body has, through neglect, been allowed to remain immobile for a long period, and the body goes into a pinched posture that is almost impossible to straighten out. It is often painful—and always sad—because it is preventable.

It is important to aim for 100, but it is even more important to aim for 100 by remaining straight. Stretch your head up and keep your chin up, knees straight, and shoulders back. Be an exclamation point!

STEP 89. Work Dem Bones

Every year, 1.2 million fractures occur in America. These busted bones often result not from big-time falls, but from rather trivial incidents. The bony girders of our bodies are simply not strong enough even for minor overloads.

The principal cause of weak bones, osteoporosis, is insufficient exercise. Certainly low calcium intake and hormonal factors also enter in, but it is the decades of underwork that are the principal villain. Ninety percent of women over 75 have osteoporosis. Two weeks in bed washes as much calcium out of the bones as an entire year's worth of aging. Bone loss is accelerated fiftyfold by forced rest.

The common wisdom is that running is bad for older people's bones and joints, particularly the knees. Not only is there no evidence of any damage to older joggers caused by the years of running, but joggers' bones, particularly the spine, are in even better shape than those of inactive people. If you don't work them bones, they are going to deteriorate and your risk of fracture will skyrocket.

Weak muscles mean weak bones. Persons who are stronger have thicker bones. It is not just the bone that is weakened by lack of use, but the muscle as well. Certainly weak bones and weak muscles go together, and together they conspire to make fractures a too-common feature in the lives of many older people. Someone calculated that the adverse combination accounts for one death every twenty minutes—and they are all preventable. The incidence of fractures doubles every five years, so by age 90 one in every three women will have broken their hips.

It has been suggested that bone loss starts in the thirties and proceeds from there, and that once it is lost, it cannot be replaced. Yet a research study at Washington University in St. Louis found that a two-year exercise program increased bone mass 6 percent in active compared to inactive older women. So, as with everything else I've discussed, it is never too late to start.

I encourage my older patients to be sure their dietary calcium intake is adequate—the equivalent of two glasses of milk per day—and I routinely encourage my women patients to take hormone replacement therapy. But it is on the area of encouraging exercise, particularly of the weight-bearing variety, that I place most emphasis. It is never too early or too late to start a preventive program of activity, even walking, to put the bones and muscles to work. The only good fractured hip or vertebra is the one that is avoided. Once a fracture occurs, not only is there substantial pain and immobility, but the entire quality of life is placed at risk.

The alternative is safe, cheap, and universally available and effective. Muscles and bones are meant to be used. The couch potato's bones are like mush, and even a minor awkward twist or turn may mean a trip to the hospital and months of misery. Stay away from fractures—move.

STEP 90. Respect Your Back

The spine is comprised of thirty-one vertebrae, arranged like children's building blocks except that they have pieces of gristle (the intervertebral discs) sitting between each of them to cushion impact. The spine stretches from the base of the skull to the sacrum and the pelvis and is the tent pole on which the organs and tissues of our chest and abdomen are suspended.

There has probably been too much attention paid to the discs and vertebrae. These are the items that appear on an X ray. But it is in the muscles, ligaments, and tendons where the main part of the story lies. With decades of couch and desk sitting, the muscles and ligaments start to sag. The vertebrae then develop too much leeway in their motion, beginning to scrape and pinch. Low back pain results.

With an acute pain, the back, like any inflamed joint, should take it easy so the inflammation can die down. Ice and analgesics are also part of the acute prescription for sore backs.

The great bulk of back distress is chronic in nature, and here is where exercise comes in. The back is like any joint, except it is really a whole series of them working together. To keep working well, it must be kept strong and flexible. Each part of it should be put through its full range of motion. The opposing muscles for the back are the abdominals, so these, too, must be kept fit. If one or the other predominates, imbalance occurs. A weak back is a sore back.

Your spine is made to be used but not abused. Sudden heavy lifting and twisting places stress on the many joints between the spinal bodies. Clearly the way to protect the spine is to keep it strong. Regular back use also protects again against osteoporosis and its frequent end product of compression fractures. These hurtful events are nearly always preventable.

The back prescription is three-times-weekly sessions of leg lifts, leg curls, and toe touches in combination.

Your back is your main pillar. It needs to carry you through your whole life journey, which means that you should buttress it with regular exercise and flexing. If you don't, it will start to ache and diminish the quality of your later years.

However, if you are smart, you will treat your back with respect and appreciation for all the good work it does for you. Reward it with regular exercise.

STEP 91. Honor Your Neck

As a doctor who takes care of a lot of old people, I see that the neck is underrecognized as a source of trouble, and therefore worth particular attention. Headaches, numb hands, and dizziness are the three main symptoms of a bum neck. Whenever I hear any of these complaints, I immediately focus my exam on the neck. The nerves and blood supply to the head and arms all run through the neck.

The neck is a series of seven small vertebrae, on the top one of which rests the skull. I compare the neck to an accordion that has a certain amount of play in it. When there is injury or inflammation, the muscles that hold the neck in place contract just like an accordion, and the nerves, muscles, and arteries get pinched. Headaches and numb hands result when the nerves are pinched, and dizziness and lightheadedness occur when the arteries are knuckled. Often these symptoms are worse in the morning, because during the night you sleep with your chin on your chest, and the neck muscles tend to gel like gelatin. As you waken and stretch out the spasm, the kinks in the nerves and arteries are relieved, and the symptoms subside.

The neck is what I call an organ of response. Think of a lioness for a moment. When she is alarmed, her neck is tight, her ears are up, her eyes stare, and her shoulders tense as she readies herself for any emergency. Your anatomy is not so obvious as the lion's, but when you are on the alert, your neck and shoulder muscles tighten, and your stare and posture are fixed and vividly attentive. In contrast, when everything is calm, you tend to hold your head in different attitudes, shifting easily and frequently, relieving tension. So the neck is a major seat of stress.

The first approach to a tight, painful neck is not a collar, traction, or referral to physical therapy, but exercise. The mischief that injuries and stress can cause your neck are well addressed by keeping your neck strong and supple. You can keep it strong by pushing your head forward and then back against your cupped palm for a count of ten alternately several times a day. You can keep it supple by gently moving it forward, backward, and sideways. Perform these exercises gently; therapists generally advise against rotating the neck.

Look at the horizon, not at the ground. Keep your chin up and in. Keep your shoulders back. Keep your head high. Stand tall. See over the hill. Be proud, look proud. Respect your neck.

STEP 92. Keep Breathing

Two hundred years ago Joseph Priestley discovered oxygen. His discovery led him to speculate that this common and vital element was both life giving and hazardous at the same time. His suspicion has proved correct. We can't live without it, but it also causes mischief along the way.

The question then immediately arises: If oxygen is a bad actor, why should you exercise, which results in breathing and puffing along the way and thereby subjects you to increased risk of oxygen-caused damage? The accelerated traffic in oxygen does result in increased generation of potentially harmful free radicals, the same free radicals that are widely held to be responsible for the deteriorating changes associated with the aging process. So does exercise accelerate aging? No!

The explanation probably resides in the fact that the systems your body has developed to get rid of these free radicals are also increased by exercise. These scavenger devices clearly go up in trained people. People with higher oxygen transport capacity (VO_2 max) not only generate more free radicals, but they also get rid of them faster.

In a sense, this system is like the old argument about heartbeats and exercise. If every heart has only so many beats in them, why use them up by exercising? Well, it is true that exercise increases pulse rate. But the resting pulse is substantially slower in fit than in unfit persons. A fit person's resting pulse is 48 instead of the usual 70. Sure, his pulse goes up to 120 or 130 during exercise, but the rest of the time it beats at a stately and efficient pace. This means that the net result is fewer beats a day.

I don't fear free radicals. I count on fitness to manage them. But what if you want a booster? Can antioxidants, such as vitamin E or vitamin C, help? There are a number of experiments in animals and people that have been designed to determine whether these compounds can either boost exercise performance or decrease oxygen damage created during exercise. The results vary, but so far there is no evidence that vitamin E improves exercise performance.

Personally I don't take antioxidant supplements, although many of my colleagues do. I am ready to be persuaded that they are of real value, but I do not feel that we yet know enough to make this blanket recommendation. On the other hand, physical exercise has multiple, unambiguous credentials as a keystone strategy in reaching 100.

STEP 93. Use Your Brain—Exercise

You know that exercise is good for your bones, your muscles, your heart, your cholesterol, etc., but what about that organ that sits between your ears, your brain? After all, your brain is you. A surgeon can transplant any other part of your body, and you would still be you. But if you received a new brain, you would become someone else.

What happens to your brain when you exercise? We know that on any exertion, blood is shifted from the unessential parts of the body—such as the intestine and kidneys—to the arms and legs, where the work is going on. The brain, however, is spared this diversion, so adequate blood supply is constantly assured. It continues to receive its pint and a half of blood every minute. As we study the evolutionary chain, the brain grows in proportion to the complexity of the movements the animal makes. Predatory animals have bigger brains than prey animals, and this brain size is associated with more intricate lifestyles. Fit people have faster nerve conduction, in accord with the "use it or lose it" principle. It makes sense, then, that the more you practice some movement, the more efficient the muscles, circulation, and nerves become.

Whatever part of the brain is involved in an activity will grow, just as a muscle does when it is used. Marian Diamond showed that Einstein's parietal lobes, the associative part, were huge. In a similar way, violinists, bakers, and car mechanics each have brains that reflect parts of the brain they use most.

Growth and development require several things: an energy flow, growth factors, circulatory support, and adequate nutrition. All of these elements are provided by exercise. Exercise prompts the release of adrenalin, a very potent brain stimulant. We are more alert when adrenalin is present; sleep occurs in its absence.

I was thrilled when I read a research paper by Bob Dustman in Salt Lake City. He selected a group of older persons and tested them before and after an exercise protocol. Not only did all the predicted other benefits ensue, but the IQs of these persons went up as well. A more recent experiment reported from North Carolina showed that a six-week brisk walking program increased the cognitive abilities of older persons 7.5 percent. Wow! Exercise increases IQ! That's something, but on reflection it makes sense that it should be true.

So we learn another benefit of an exercise program. It is reported that smart people exercise more. Do they exercise because they are smart, or are they smart because they exercise? As you age, you are at risk for loss of brain power. Most of this loss is not due to age, but is instead the result of pulling back from the business of being fully alive. Think, move, think, move. Your brain will thank you for it.

STEP 94. Chase the Blues

Movement is good for you. Every organ, tissue, and cell in your body works better when it is active. Movement is good for your body, and it is good for your spirit. Even thinking about movement makes you feel brighter. A frolicking colt, a tumbling puppy, a romping child bring smiles. It is hard to conceive of feeling bad after a roller-coaster ride, downhill ski run, or merry-go-round spin. A jet plane, race car, or speedboat creates excitement. Movement is an upper.

Sitting is a downer. For a long time there has been a suspected relationship between inactivity and depression. The very idea of a caged animal is depressing, but as I've said before, all of us are zoo animals. Our culture has placed us in inactivity cages. Maybe the only ones who aren't depressed are those of us who are active. It has been asserted that no depression can withstand a ten-mile run. Psychologists and psychiatrists have embraced the notion that physical exercise is an important form of therapy for depressed people.

How could exercise help depression? The chemical modulator of the many body adaptations that accompany physical exercise is adrenalin. One of the various effects of adrenalin is to act as a stimulus for the release of endorphins in the brain. The endorphins are chemicals that nature has created to make us pain insensitive. The evolutionary advantage to being resistant to pain, while engaged in the survival strategy of fight or flight, is obvious. Wounds don't hurt until the battle is over. A fellow ran almost the entire Boston Marathon with a broken leg. He didn't feel it until the race was over. Together, adrenalin and endorphins are uppers. Depressed people have less of both. The preferred way of treating depression is to restore the deficiency in adrenalin and endorphins. Nature's way is prescribing exercise.

As you dare to be 100, losses occur along the way. Being physically fit allows you better to bear the burden those losses thrust upon you. There is an inevitable tendency to slow down as you age; the very thought of having to keep up with the trail of grandchildren is daunting. But the better able you are to do it, the less chance you will have of becoming depressed. The last of life should not be lived with a sad expression. It should be lived with a bright and optimistic outlook. A physical exercise program is a central part of maintaining that attitude. A walk to the store, library, or post office is better medicine than anything I have in my black bag.

STEP 95. Be Sexy, Be Fit

As sex is identified as a major quality-of-life issue, it is appropriate to inquire whether being physically fit enhances late-life sexuality. There have been only a few studies that addressed the topic. Dr. Jim White at the University of California in San Diego selected ninety-five sedentary middle-aged men, who exercised briskly for one hour 3 times a week for nine months. Those men who worked hardest at the workouts reported more frequent sexual activity, a more reliable function during sex, and a higher percentage of quality orgasm. The control group reported no such changes. No pain, no gain.

The penis is a vascular organ. Exercise is a potent stimulator of circulation (although erections during physical activity would seem unlikely). Exercise is an effective technique in correcting erectile difficulties. How much of the benefit derives from a tune-up of the vascular system and how much derives from an increased sense of self-esteem (the active exercise group also lost 19 percent of body fat) is unknown. But everyone acknowledges that the brain is the most important sex organ. Anything that improves the brain's image of self is bound to improve sexuality.

Several years ago my son Walter and I did a survey of the sex habits of the men over 70 who belong to the Fifty-Plus Fitness Association. Of thirty-eight members, average age 75, 58 percent still rated their sex lives as good or very good, another 23 percent fair, and only 19 percent reported their sex lives as poor. Kinsey's original 1948 report recorded that 55 percent of 75-year-old men were impotent. Our small survey would indicate that an active group does far better.

What about women? It is clear that physical exercise is a wonderful assistance to some of the changes associated with menopause. Fitness evens out many of the bumps and also adds immeasurably to older women's sense of confidence, health, and independence. For a large number of women, the quality of their sexual lives improves after menopause. Being physically fit helps. Exercise mandates a continued body awareness, which is a further health and sex benefit. Continued engagement in all aspects of healthful living leads to good sex.

Good sex is good for your health. Good health is good for your sexuality.

Be fit and sexy—hopefully until 100.

STEP 96. Avoid the Big C—Exercise

Does taking a walk help prevent cancer? There is increasing evidence that cancer is not just a random event—that it really has a strong relationship to how we live our lives. The linkage between cigarette smoking and lung and bladder cancers is the prime example. But if it is so obvious that how we live causes cancer, isn't there similar evidence that how we live helps to prevent it? Yes.

More and more researchers are finding that physical fitness helps us prevent cancer. No one suggests that being fit eliminates the risk of cancer altogether, but numerous studies strikingly illustrate lower rates of the disease in people who exercise. Some forms of cancer seem particularly responsive to an active lifestyle, colon cancer among them. It has been known for some time that the length of time it takes food to transit your intestinal tract from entrance to exit is considerably shorter in active people. Without question, diet, too, has a lot to do with cancer. The inference, then, is that if some cancer-provoking material stays in contact with the lining of the colon for longer, it provides an increased risk of colon cancer. Whether this is the explanation for its protective role or not is uncertain, but the lower rate of colon cancer in active people is unassailable.

The other principal types of malignancy that have been shown to react to an actively lived life are the reproductive organ cancers: breast, uterus, and ovary for the women, and prostate for men. The possible mechanism behind such protection is the same for both sexes, involving a lowering of tissue exposure to levels of the sex hormones estrogen and testosterone. For women it is clear, particularly in those young elite athletes whose menstrual patterns are disrupted by their intense pursuit of fitness, that fitness and low body fat content dramatically lower estrogen levels. Consequently, those organs that are targets for estrogen will not be bathed in decades of higher estrogen amounts and consequently have less potential for malignancy.

For men, the story is the same. Exercise lowers testosterone levels, and the prostate is clearly sensitive to testosterone. Men with prostate cancer have been reported to have higher levels of testosterone than others. Often the first treatment for prostate cancer that has spread is castration. Such a step drops testosterone levels virtually to zero and frequently results in a marked reduction of the spread of the tumor. If your prostate gland is exposed to a lower testosterone level over the lifetime, the risk decreases dramatically. Other cancers, such as lung cancer, are also low in fit persons, but this is felt to be due to the fact that few fit people smoke.

Cancer is such an evil villain that I feel every one of us should be doing everything we can to prevent it. Cure is still too rare, so prevention is vital. Being physically fit has excellent credentials as a vaccine we should all be using regularly.

STEP 97. Walk Away from Infection

As with resistance to cancer, fitness also provides protection against infection. The ability to ward off the threats posed by the sea of bacteria and viruses in which we live is dependent on elaborate and still not totally understood mechanisms. In the last ten years we have discovered dozens of body chemicals that protect us, and physical exercise has been shown to provide higher levels of many of these defense compounds. Fit people get colds less often. The Center for Disease Control in Atlanta found that those persons who jogged 25 miles a week had one or two respiratory infections per year compared to the general index population of three per year.

Of course, it was also found that 13 percent of the people who ran in the Boston Marathon in 1987 came down with flu or cold within a week of the race, compared with only 2 percent of the spectators. British Olympic gold medalist Sebastian Coe failed to qualify for the 1988 games because of a debilitating cold. Why? Overtraining not only fails to increase resistance to infection, but it also probably lowers it.

How does exercise increase immunity? The link is not fully established, but we do know that physical exercise is accompanied by an outpouring of adrenalin, the compound that makes the heart pump faster and produce sweating and metabolic adaptations such as high blood sugar. It also makes the body temperature go up, such as during infection. Adrenalin causes the spleen to release immune substances and the number of infection-fighting white blood cells to go up as well. It is also possible that adrenalin provides benefit to allergy sufferers as well. Many allergy medications have as their primary ingredient adrenalin or a related compound.

When exercise is extreme, however, the stress state results. As noted earlier, stress is accompanied by higher levels of cortisone. Cortisone, unlike adrenalin, produces a decreased resistance to infection, and potentially the component that puts competitors straining at the edge of their abilities at risk.

A clear marker of older people is a reduced immune response. But we must ask again whether the decreased response is due to aging or inactivity. We haven't recruited enough 100-year-old athletes to answer this question definitively, but it seems likely that the reason older persons seem prone to infection is that they are often frail—not only in bone and muscle, but in antibody response as well. The logical proposition, then, is to offset the supposed decline in resistance to infection as we age. You need to retain fitness over the lifetime, not as a weekend warrior who puts yourself constantly at risk by overdoing and putting a stress on your body systems, but with a planned, regular exercise program in which all body systems participate in a meaningful way.

This does not mean that you should continue to exercise when you are really sick with an infection. If you have fever or general symptoms such as muscle or headaches, you should lie low for a few days. But don't let a runny nose alone interrupt your active lifestyle.

STEP 98. Know That Aging Is Incurable

Five years ago the wire services were clogged with reports that human growth hormone, as advocated by a group of workers at the University of Wisconsin, was the answer to the deteriorations of aging. I cringe when I hear such news, because I know that soon the phone will be jangling with crowds of patients wanting to get on the bandwagon. To this day, I see advertisements in popular magazines of clinics near or below the Mexican border where rejuvenation therapy with a youth hormone (HGH) is provided. Such ballyhoo is not unique. Youth farms have flourished for centuries, largely in Europe, where flocks of the hopeful converge in the search for renewed energies and childhood retrieved.

Like other schemes, rejuvenation therapy has some rationale behind it. Certainly muscle strength is lower in older people, and this muscle weakness translates into bundles of clinical problems. It is also true that older people have lower levels of growth hormones in the blood than younger people. Hence the suggestion that restoration of HGH levels to normal will restore the lost strength of youth.

It now appears that growth hormone use is loaded with problems. The important research group at Washington University in St. Louis reported their experience with HGH in older people. Half of their group of subjects stopped the use of the treatment within two to eight weeks of its initiation, due to symptoms of arthritis and fluid retention. This high percentage of side effects occurred despite low doses of the drug. Further, those subjects who were able to complete four months of treatment failed to exhibit substantial increases in muscle strength. Other reports of side effects secondary to growth hormone use include induction of diabetes and cancer.

The reason older people's muscles grow weak and their HGH levels are low is not due to the fact that they are old. Their muscles are weak and their hormone levels are low because they have stopped exercising. The answer to this problem lies not at the drugstore but in the walk to and from the drugstore. Such treatment is effective, safe, devoid of side effects, and cheap. HGH treatment costs in the range of $15,000 per year.

Nevertheless, Americans seem destined to continue to

seek salvation in a pill bottle. Technology appeals to us. Easy-fix solutions are part of our culture, but muscles don't yet know that. The way to keep older muscles fit is to use them, not jack them up with anabolic steroids.

It is still possible that growth hormone injections may have a useful role in medical care, such as following a severe injury or stroke, but your aging remains yours to manage, with little help on the horizon from your friendly pharmacist. To keep your growth hormone levels up and your bones and your muscles strong, start by taking a walk.

STEP 99. You Don't Have to Win

One of the treasures of my life was my friendship with George Sheehan. We ran together, joked together, philosophized together. His wonderful writing nourished me. His view of the integration of exercise and living was brilliant, and his book *Running and Being* remains one of my top favorites. George died after a long bout with prostate cancer. We talked often toward the end. He was a terrible patient, as most doctors are. I did my best to keep his spirits and energy up.

We were soul brothers except for one thing. George wanted to win. His life strategy was to be first. Probably not as intense as Vince Lombardi's, his insistence in beating the other fellow was nevertheless a constant. In contrast, my ego survives being passed by all the time. It doesn't bother me one bit to come in last, as long as I come in. I love the saying "Life is the one game you win by coming in last." I am practicing that approach.

My analysis of exercise is to pay no attention to time. The rest of my life is so driven by fifteen-minute increments that when I jog or do any exercise, I want to do it without having to finish in any particular time. Who is going to remember who came in first anyway?

The idea of competition and winning is part of the lure of

sports for many people, but it is also a major barrier for others. In competing, the likelihood of losing—after all, there can be only one winner, and a whole lot of losers—is intimidating and therefore a negative feature in encouraging people to exercise. But exercise isn't about winning. It is about participating, doing something, anything.

The process of aging, slow as it is, dictates that you are going to lose if you insist on competing with the you of yesterday. Yet you can be the best for today by being active and retaining your best function and form.

The need for physical exercise is a remnant of millions of years of walking. Such a pace has sustained our existence on this earth, and it is how we came to understand our surroundings. In our lifelong journey, speed and winning have little relevance. Being a part of nature—not dominating it—is the issue.

But just because the idea of winning is not the reason for exercise, it doesn't mean that you can sit around and watch. Someone wisely said that life is not a spectator sport. It has to be played and engaged. Growing older is a slow process, but it can become much faster if you don't participate. The difference between activity and inactivity, when multiplied by years of living, is the major determinant of how your later life will be lived. If you race at the start and don't pace yourself, you will lose. If you don't even start—or halt along the way—you will lose. Keeping the pace, staying the course, is the master strategy. If you offered me fast, first, strong, or steady, I would always choose steady.

STEP 100. Just Do It

Okay, I lied. There aren't just ninety-nine steps to 100. In fact, the hundredth step sums up all the others.

Golf, like bowling, is a wonderful recreation, but it just isn't enough push to qualify as quality exercise. To do my body good, movement must have some pace to it. Walking is clearly the form of exercise that is most universally available and could be a boon to our nation's fitness profile—if we would only remember individually and collectively how to walk. As it is now, we cluster around elevators to go up one floor. The airport is also a challenge—when an escalator, horizontal or vertical, is available, nearly everyone uses it. Stairs become nearly obsolete. In public buildings, they are often built in unfriendly corners where rubbish accumulates. I would favor prohibiting elevators for ascents of fewer than six floors.

Other athletic endeavors, such as tennis, basketball, baseball, football, biking, skiing, etc., are all qualified by how the sport is played. I know tennis players who are either so skillful or so lazy that they rarely move from the center of the court. Other sports are the same. If you play with a level of intensity that causes the heart to pound and the breath to pant, that's when health benefits accrue. But even some football players are in lousy shape. Just being strong isn't enough. You can be strong as a bull and still be in poor condition. I delight in the stories of body builders who flunk the physical exams for such-and-such a job position because they are in poor condition.

To be successful, an exercise program should have an element of recreation and renewal in it. Exercising just because it is good for you isn't enough for most people. It should be fun, too. If the exercise is perceived as work, chances are you won't sustain it. For some people this means group activities, for others it means a solo experience. For some it must be done in the morning, for others the evening. There are lots and lots of ways to be fit.

But be more than body fit, be whole person fit—body, mind, spirit all in harmony, balance, vitality. This is the ideal. It takes guts and smarts. It takes involvement.

The key is to do it, just do it.

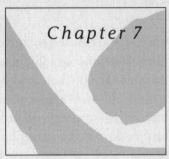

Chapter 7

Asked the great Sage, Satchel Paige,
"Do you really know your time—
Are you over the hump, in your last slump,
Or maybe still in your prime?"

Know Your Age—Act Your Age

Satch's immortal question "How old would you be if you didn't know how old you were?" has been pondered for thousands of years by poets, philosophers, scholars, physicians, actuaries, public policy makers, and everybody else. It doesn't take much imagination to realize that the date on your birth certificate gives only a rough estimate of how old you really are. As to what really matters, how you feel and how you are functioning are the keys. Are you a go-go, slo-go, or no-go? Someone suggested that we ought to record our time from the end backwards, as in a football or basketball game—how much time do we still have left, rather than how much time we have lived. Obviously, of course, none of us has had a good handle on when we were going to die. But what if you could know with some confidence the date on which your life policy would expire?

What is your age gauge? How old are you really? How many grains of sand are left in your hourglass? The word that has been coined to explore this idea is "biomarker." A biomarker is supposed to be a test that can give a good indication, not just of chronologic age, but more importantly of biological age. If you had a good biomarker, or a set of them, it would help you make some significant decisions. If we only had an age gauge, like a meat thermometer, that we could insert somewhere to see how "done" we were, we'd be ahead of where we are now. The tests we now perform in a doctor's office—blood pressure, cholesterol level, electrocardiogram, and the rest—are almost worthless to Satchel's question. Substantial scientific effort is being expended to explore and establish valid biomarkers. Most of the changes commonly associated with old people are really not dependent on the passage of time; they result mostly from disuse. As you might imagine, this mislabeling leads to all sorts of wrong judgments.

Think of your car. You know the date you bought it and how many miles it has run. Is this what matters? What if it were a lemon right out of the factory, imperfectly made, and in trouble almost as soon as you bought it? Certainly, then, the car's age is not the issue. What if you or your teenage son had a substantial accident with the car, resulting in major damage to the body's frame or engine? Similarly, the car's failure to function perfectly cannot be blamed on the fact that it's old. But what if the car was well made, and it encountered no accidents along its route, but you put bad gas in it, left it exposed to harsh weather, didn't lubricate it, or in other ways neglected its maintenance? Well, obviously it will start to malfunction, because of lack of preventive care.

How well an old car runs is therefore the result of all three of these elements: faulty manufacture, misadventure, and poor maintenance. What kind of a test can you, or a prospective secondhand buyer, perform to assure that the car will demonstrate continued good performance? What are the automarkers of an old car? As a car ignoramus, about all I would know to do is to check the tire tread and the speedometer reading. (That's why I don't buy secondhand cars—I have no faith in my ability to read the automarkers.)

It is recognized that it is not how the car looks that matters, but how it runs. We all know stories of the secondhand heap that is gleamingly polished but can't make it out of the lot. In other words, it is not how old you are that counts, it's how you are old.

The new interest spawned by the growth of the health maintenance organizations (HMOs) is in risk assessment. This is another reframing of Satchel Paige's question. "What are the risks that will stand in your way in reaching 100?" Certain obvious issues emerge. Some are structural, some are functional, some are due to genetic factors, some to lightning, but most are due to dissonance, or poor health maintenance. This is fundamentally a good-news story, because both accidents and dissonance can be avoided.

We desperately need tools that are helpful in predicting where the trouble spots are likely to emerge. We must get out of the habit of waiting until the body springs a leak or otherwise breaks down before the system kicks in. In my view, we now have enough smarts to be able to craft new approaches that will avoid the very expensive and often futile high-tech efforts that define much of present-day medicine. We must look at the whole person—not just his or her parts—and over a period of time, not just a single moment. And last, we must look at the person in a social context, not just as someone isolated from the rest of the world.

It is obvious that much effort has gone into the task of answering Satchel's question, "How old are you really?" The task is a regular part of my job of taking care of old people in my medical office. All of my patients want to know how they are doing and what they could do to do better. They are asking, "What is my lifetime?

NEW AGE TEST

It is time to propose a New Age Test. This test acknowledges the new understandings and realities I've addressed in this book. It uses physical, psychological, and sociological guidelines. It acknowledges that we are elastic and mightily capable of change and growth and repair, even into old age. The new test is optimistic.

To establish the new age test, the first task is to assess what your body does. My explorations reveal three primary tasks that the human organism pursues: It moves, it thinks, and it makes love. It is true the body does other things, too—it eats, breathes, and excretes—but these functions pretty much act to support the basic three above.

First, movement. No one can dispute the fundamental role of movement that nature has assigned our bodies. On a mass basis, most of our energy is focused on getting from one place to another. Our muscles and bones are our vehicles. Our circulatory, nervous, and digestive systems serve mobility. Movement is a central theme in all of nature, and it is no less so with us, although we seem to be failing in this job, due to our relatively recent cultural laziness.

Second, cognition. We honor ourselves with the label "sapiens." It is our distinction. Other creatures outperform us in virtually all other categories of life, but intelligence is our crowning glory. The body's mechanics ensure that under all sorts of challenge—hot, cold, infection, starvation, extreme exertion—the brain is protected first, then the other organs get what's left over.

Third, sex. Many biologists would claim reproduction is the only purpose for all of nature, that each of us is only a temporary organization of flesh or plant stuff, the duty of which is to transmit genetic information down through time. I identify sex in a much less restrictive manner, proposing that it transcends the mere reproductive element. To me, our sexuality is one of the major life-quality issues, not confined at all to the early phases of life. Famous gerontologist Alex Comfort made perhaps his greatest contribution by emphasizing *The Joy of Sex* as we grow older. Sex is renewal, engagement, self-esteem, staying awake in life, sense preserving and extending. It provides a richness that lasts a lifetime. Comfort wrote, "Aging abolishes neither the need nor the capacity for sexual experiences."

Having asserted that movement, cognition, and sex are the three fundamental life activities, and that they remain significant throughout life, the New Age Test proceeds. You receive one point a day when you walk a mile, one point when you read a book, and one point when you make love. You can't receive more than one point for each category (if you walk two miles, for example, read two books, or make love twice); one point per day is the maximum. Each category also has equivalents: Biking, swimming, gardening, etc., count as well. Similarly, writing, playing a musical instrument, exploring on the computer, or doing crossword puzzles all count for a point. Equivalents for making love are harder to extrapolate, but they invariably involve putting your sensual self in action.

These three activities add up to a potential three-point day and twenty-one point week. At the age of 30, it's easy to say that many or most of us could come up with a number of fifteen- to twenty-point weeks. As life proceeds, however, the weekly total tends to lessen—although it shouldn't. As you focus on the three Ss of successful aging—strong, smart, and sexy—you will increase your chances of hitting the maximum point score.

Such an accounting involves your physical self. But any age test must also involve some evaluation of meaning. What is a high physical point total if life doesn't have merit? The biology of being human is necessary but insufficient.

Each of you must inevitably derive your reason for living for yourself. In my personal effort to identify my reason, my

Grandpa Bortz's exhortation "Make yourself necessary" comes closest to providing me some valid sense of why being alive matters. Albert Einstein expressed this sentiment somewhat differently:

From the standpoint of daily life, there is one thing we do know; that man is here for the sake of other men—above all, for those upon whose smile and well-being our own happiness depends and also for the countless unknown souls with whose fate we are concerned by a bond of sympathy. Many times a day I realize how my own outer and inner life is built upon the labors of my fellow men, both living and dead, and how earnestly I must exert myself in order to give in return as much as I have received.

Whatever your measure of life meaning happens to be, you receive another two points each day for pursuing that meaning. Your two-point allotment depends on your sense of being involved in life. These two points then combine with the others to make five-point days and thirty-five-point weeks. Once again, these point totals are not age sensitive. They apply over the entire lifespan. If you presume that at age 30 you are at your highest potential life energy, fully equipped with the machinery of living a rich life, that means you have seventy years more until 100, or 127,750 points.

My New Age Test provides a measure against which you can determine how successfully you approach your aging versus the usual patterns. Usual means a 2 percent loss per year versus the ideal of only 0.5 percent per year. The difference between these two is determined by your point total. If you move, think, make love, and pursue life meaning, you will continue to receive points at a high rate. You will be successful.

Using the weekly point total and the notion of usual versus successful aging, various scales emerge—the chances of living to 100, percentage likelihood, rate of aging, etc. This system provides a whole projection of how we can view and reliably predict our chances of a long, viable life.

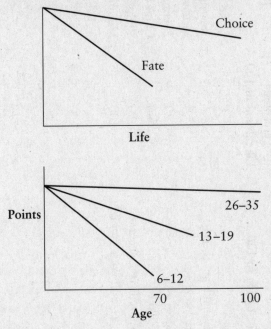

FIG. 10. Life/Fate Choice.

The difference in slope is the difference between Fate (0–20 points) and Choice (>20 points).

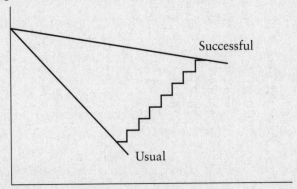

FIG. 11. 99 Steps to Successful Aging.

New Aging Test

Points per Week	Chances of Living to 100	Percentage Likelihood of 100	Rate of Aging
0–5	You're dead now	0	Gone
6–12	You'll be lucky to make another 10	1	Sinking fast
13–19	Slim; 70 is a more likely goal	5	Modest downdrift
20–25	You've got a chance	20	Average
26–30	A long, full life is likely	60	Gains offset losses
31–34	Your daily daring predicts success	90	Slight
35	A sure bet—you seize all your moments	100	Minimal

Chapter 6 provides ninety-nine action steps (and one battle cry) that lead from the steep, slippery slope of a low-point total (usual aging, disuse, and disengagement) to a high-point total (successful, active aging).

If you smoke or are otherwise self-destructive, don't bother with the test.

What remains is to determine whether you can catch up if you fall behind in your point total. The renewal capacity of the human organism is vast. This resilience aspect has yet to be explored, but the chances are that redemptive capacity exists in all of us. The essential point remains that the higher your weekly total of points, the higher your life total of points, and the greater are your chances of making 100.

Until recently, fate had decreed that you would die around age 70. Now, with the identity of elements that contribute and shape your whole life, you can track and control your biomarkers. Matters of fate have become matters of choice. Keep your point total up. Dare to be 100.

The person who dies with the most points wins.

Chapter 8

The Portrait of a Life

"You can't do that. No one knows what a whole life looks like."

"They will when we get through."

Carl Sagan exclaimed that understanding is a form of ecstasy. Ours is the first generation in the history of our species privileged enough to feel the ecstasy that derives from a deep comprehension of the dimension and dynamics of a whole lifespan.

Our parents and their parents and parents back to the beginning of time were born, lived, and died without having looked into a reflecting surface that revealed the totality of their existence. They glimpsed life as a series of isolated moments, felt the pangs of instants of pain and pleasure, and endured the defeats and glories with little if any sense of endurability, because life itself was so uncertain, short, and constantly threatened by forces and events where prayer and shamans were the sole recourse. Until now the meaning of life was sternly coded by the simple message "Stay alive."

For hundreds of thousands of generations, natural force tossed humans around like ping-pong balls in a hurricane. We created myths and religions to help sort out the uncertainties of our world. We were ignorant and passive. Here today and gone tomorrow. Nature is a neutral spectator in human affairs, indeed to all affairs. Through prior history, beneficence blends with agony to render any sense of order obscure. Millions of species arose and disappeared with no noble epitaphs to mourn their passing.

Our species has only recently arrived on the Earth scene, and is much younger than innumerable more humble creatures. Any discriminating analysis of our human nature till now would reveal that most of us are lazy and selfish, many are mean spirited, and all are shortsighted. The randomness of our lives is in most respects indistinguishable from the animal stock from which we evolved. In caves, tents, and lean-tos, our forebears wakened daily to the uncertainty of survival itself. Starvation was a constant issue. Countless ancestors were the food of other stronger and faster animals. Yet out of the crude dusts of prehistory emerge our contemporary selves, finally equipped with a sufficient fund of intellectual competence to separate us from the rest of nature. But intelligence is the most powerful insurance policy for survivability. We may have just now crossed this threshold.

A detailed assessment of the process of a human life would inevitably conclude that it is grossly misdesigned. Kierkegaard noted that life must be understood backwards, but must be lived forward. In response, Bernie Siegel proposes that since life is backwards, it makes much more sense in reverse: Death is a fundamental annoyance and should be addressed, dealt with, and therefore finished with first. Then old age is kind of a drag and tough, so we should get it over with while we are still vigorous. Then the retirement years can be pretty much fun, a reward for getting the unpleasant parts of life out of the way. Then comes the work and child-rearing time of life, which is the really important period when big things happen. Then comes adolescence and the freedom and excitements that it brings. Then comes childhood with the giggles and innocence—still more fun. Then comes infancy, with its snuggles, warmth, and serenity. Being in utero, which follows, is as comfortable as a person can possibly get. And finally comes conception and the creative fervor of two pairs of bright eyes. The lyrics of a song, "Rock Me to Sleep, Mother," written in 1860 by Elizabeth Akers Allen went "Backward, turn backward, oh time in thy flight, and make me a child again just for tonight." Well, Siegel's redesign of life is a delight, but implementing it seems to present a number of problems.

So it appears we are stuck with the present sequence. The splendor of the whole has been hidden behind the artifacts of premature death. Now with the real prospect of living our entire lives in confidence and knowledge comes the opportunity to escape the helplessness and hopelessness with which eons of fate have oppressed the lives of all before our time.

We become whole only by becoming old—only then do we develop swelling clarity. Dying young represents an incompletion. As John Bradshaw said, "Only in the evening can you know the whole day." Now we can and should grow old. Now we can know the whole of life. We need to live long enough to find out who we really are. Life is a voyage toward one's true self. With age we come closer to truth.

Knowing how to set our life clocks is a precious gift. Imagine our world if all calendars and clocks and temporal cues were removed. I must consult my watch fifty times each day. But even worse, what if all our clocks were wrong? What if we felt it was much later than it really was? We'd be eating dinner in the morning, quitting work way too soon, and looking for the end of the day when it was only partially spent, expecting midnight in the afternoon.

Having determined with confidence the human lifespan provides knowledge about the width of the canvas on which we can paint our self-portrait. Until recently the canvas size was uncertain, usually much narrower than it had to be. Now we know. I wrote earlier how Mother was confused and embarrassed by being 95. She didn't accept or play the role well. She didn't know how wide her canvas was. Knowing with some confidence that detail makes personal inventory along the way more meaningful: We know how much of the width of the canvas is covered, and we know how much is left. Several years ago, as I passed 60, I looked into the mirror to see what it was like to be 60—I hadn't been 60 before. I liked what I saw. I was healthy, had a wonderful wife and family, grandchildren, a beautiful home, a gratifying medical practice, great friends. I'd seen the world. The image that looked back at me was in great shape—better even than ten years before, with more grandkids, more experiences and perspectives, more in the savings account, new friends, new books read. I found that 60 was richer than 50, which was richer than 40, and so on.

In an op ed essay in the *New York Times*, Tom Brokaw reported his self-analysis on his 50th birthday morning.

At 50 you're no longer young. You no longer can play the part of the brash young man making the daring moves secure within the knowledge that if they don't work out there will probably be other chances. Achievement is not a cause of praise, it is expected. Suddenly all those casual promissory notes of years gone by are overdue. When we are in our 20s and 30s life's learning curve is steep but exhilarating. In our 40s we move into a cruising speed, navigating curves with the comforting knowledge that we have been through most of them before. So doesn't it follow that in the 50s you can switch to autopilot guided by stored wisdom and maturity, snapping off just the right decision or advice on matters large and small? It is finally time to be a real grown-up. Not true.

Tom went on to reflect that his father died at 69, only nineteen years further on, yielding a "hardening realization of mortality."

These, then, are visions at 60 and 50. The album shots are

interesting, but of far greater import are the shots ten years from then, at 70, 80, and beyond. On what will these next images depend? Certainly our status checks will not reveal a progressive improvement if we go onto autopilot, if we allow our weekly point totals to droop. It depends on guts and smarts. We are in charge of our futures. The clock keeps ticking away. The challenge is to jam as much meaning as possible into the intervals between the clicks.

This part of drawing the first accurate portrait of life has focused on its length, its horizontal quantifiable dimensions. But everyone would agree that having only this aspect is incomplete. The more important part of the story involves the qualitative aspects of life. With what do we fill in the portrait of life? What colors, textures, contexts, mixtures, curves, and other shapes of innumerable size and contour? To attempt an analysis of the elements that give life its quality, I suggest two broad categories of criteria, A and B, roughly reciprocal of one another. Group A elements are those of early life; Group B are those of late life. The list of words on page 257 reveals my choices. You should modify it to reflect your values and insights. Early-in-life qualities that predominate are basically narcissistic, reflecting a self-centered materialistic and time-urgent life pattern. "What's in it for me?"

"I want what I want and I want it right now!" "Never trust anyone over 30." Personal rights, nonconformity, and adventurism are paramount.

Conversely, old age offers the opposite: devotion, externally centered, and time and material insensitive. I have witnessed many, many times old patients who have little or no interest in personal possessions. Time, too, loses its pressuring impact toward the end of life. A heightened sense of responsibility should and often does occur as life progresses. Peter Laslett, the eminent British historian, notes the appropriateness of increased responsibility with aging—a youngster has not yet lived long enough to have had much impact on his or her surroundings, whereas a 70- or 80-year-old has had many decades to be acting on the world, conforming it to one's actions, and thus the increased responsibility that accompanies aging.

A Christmas morning gives evidence of the reciprocal nature of these various qualities. The grandkids are in mad pursuit of as much possession as they can accumulate. The success of their day depends on the size of the pile. On the

LIFE ELEMENTS

A. Early	B. Late
Randomness	Selectivity
Chaos	Order
Appearance	Significance
Things	Ideas
Time urgent	Timeless
Me	You
Being	Becoming
Fact	Content
Rights	Responsibilities
Tangible	Intangible
Simplicity	Complexity
Intolerant	Tolerant
Judgmental	Forgiving
Categorical	Shadings
Instinct	Conscience
Impatient	Patient
Certainty	Uncertainty
Abrupt	Steady
Restless	Peaceful
Strength	Skill
Receiving	Giving
Selfish	Generous
Structure	Function

other hand, older participants in the festivities derive the most pleasure from seeing the interaction of others and from new experiences and opportunities granted by tickets, books, or other carefully considered gifts. The more successful a person is in shifting strategies, the more competent and complete will be the last part of the portrait.

There are, of course, infinite combinations of elements from lists A and B throughout life, yet there are reciprocal relationships that are commonly found, and these are in a way biomarkers in themselves. Figure 12 shows an attempt to create a life portrait.

But this interpretation is not complete enough. It neglects vital and defining parts of life's transitions and developments. Figure 13 incorporates some of these. First are the downward lines of aging, the commonly observed physical, intellectual, and emotional changes as the years pass. As documented earlier, these changes are real and without challenge, but the acuteness of their decline depends to a large measure on how we live our lives. If we live forcefully and successfully, this decline is only ½ percent per year. If we abandon ourselves to noninvolvement, the slope can be much steeper. Conversely, virtually at birth education and knowledge begin to increase, hopefully over the entirety of the lifespan. Coupled with knowledge, and certainly part of its creation, is a widening experience. It must be noted that adversity and defeat are experiences that provide sturdier gains in knowledge than ease and lack of challenge.

As a byproduct of knowledge and experience comes usefulness. As I've said previously, being useful is, for me, our identifying purpose in life. And as Ben Franklin asked, "Of what use is a newborn baby?" In my 60s I believe I am a more useful being than I was forty or twenty or even five years ago. This is an endorsement of life process. If I found myself less useful, I would inevitably question what I am still doing here.

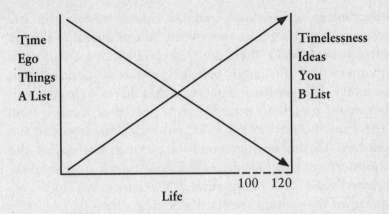

FIG. 12. Life Components.

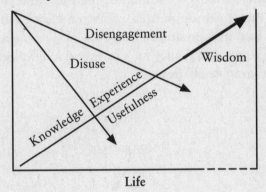

FIG. 13. Life Forces.

As life's increasing trajectory of years proceeds, the pinnacle intellectual achievement is that of gaining wisdom, mankind's highest possession.

Yet these upward vectors of time direction are not assured. They are a choice. They take smarts and guts to assert. A common pattern of a life portrait cut short is seen in figure 14 on the next page. The early and midlife patterns sustain, but shortly after midlife a profound vector change occurs. Both direction and energy veer from the upward course. Disengagement occurs. Such common change is seen over and over again and happens shortly after the midpoint of the full life course. Usually there are triggers, losses of one type or another—job loss, family role loss, spouse loss, sexual loss, economic loss—whatever acts to signal that it is time to hunker down, go from forward gear to neutral or reverse, from active involvement to autopilot, surrender of autonomy and mastery. This moment changes the portrait. Carl Sagan and Anne Druyan conclude their book *Shadows of Forgotten Ancestors* with this observation: "Our ancestors have bequeathed us—within certain limits to be sure—the ability to change our institutions and ourselves. Nothing is preordained . . . Maturity entails a readiness, painful and wrenching though it may be, to look squarely into the long dark places, into the fearsome shadows. In this act of ancestral remembrance and acceptance may be found a light by which to see our children safely home."

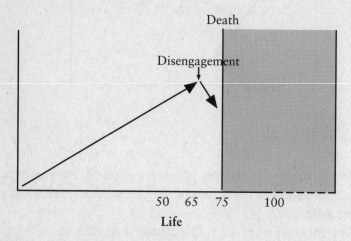

FIG. 14. Present Life Portrait.

It is no coincidence that 75 is the median age of death in America. It follows predictably from the time of disengagement. It is nature's confirmation that when meaning becomes lost, life is over. Too often death occurs after the third quarter, at nine o'clock, after the third act of a four-act play, or when the portrait is only three-fourths finished. Life is about choices all along the line, but particularly at that midpoint when a "go, no-go" decision is required. When "no" becomes an easier answer than "yes," when pessimism wins out over optimism, when loss overcomes possible gain, then life and its full expression are in jeopardy. Matters of fate become matters of choice. The most critical choice is that of staying involved, giving life its full play.

If and when you decide to make the choice, then you will have responded with guts to the dare. You will have the opportunity to live your whole life and explore its further reach. Death will become irrelevant.

As you sustain your purpose, courage, and involvement, life proceeds to its inevitable and logical end. Having given everything away, possessions lose all significance, time isn't about rushing, and death loses its sting. Personal needs will be ful-

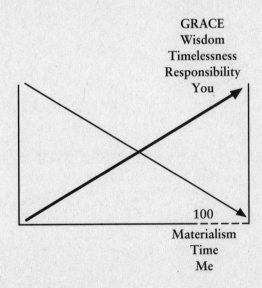

FIG. 15. Ideal Life Portrait.

filled, and your communion with what truly matters will be complete. You will therefore be invested in immortality. All of the ego elements of youth have been transformed to the externalities of cosmic order and good. Your plan is complete. You achieve grace.

By exploiting the simple earnest effort of living a full and engaged existence, the state of grace appears as the defined reward, not as an anointing for a saintly deed or heroic act, but the logical end product of the good life. The life portrait, drawn by our hand, is complete. This moment emerges as one of the most iridescent in all history. For the first time, we can draw ourselves.

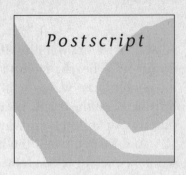

Postscript

Life has an end. Its end needs its own order, rationality, and dignity. I have spent much time pondering my own end, and this is what I see.

As the end approaches, I choose to become a beach-comber. This claim may sound whimsical or maybe silly, but it is not. It is highly considered and deliberate. To take to the beach at the end of life makes a lot of sense if you pause to think about it.

First, it is cheap and requires almost no worldly goods to support. I have earlier stated my intention of divesting myself of every possession as life closes. I feel no debt of gratitude to the IRS for their gentle shepherding through life, and I choose passionately to leave nothing for them to pick over.

But beyond the material advantage provided by a beach, it offers central others. My careful analysis of why many people are forced to seek institutional care at the end of life yields three reasons: immobility, incontinence, and cognitive impairment. Buried somewhere in these three diagnoses is the explanation for why each such individual is now in a nursing home. I choose not to require this support. The beach is the answer. First, immobility. If I have trouble moving and fall down on a beach, I won't hurt myself. Secondly, if I am incontinent, the waves will wash it away. Thirdly, if I act a little batty on the beach, it's okay, because I'm supposed to act that way on a beach anyway.

And finally, when the final swoon comes, the high tide will take me out to sea, where life all began in the first place.

Further Reading

Age and Structural Lag edited by Mathilda Riley, Robert Kahn, and Ann Foner, John Wiley, 1994.

At Home in the Universe by Stuart Kaufman, Oxford University Press, 1992.

The Biology of Life Span by Leonid Gavrilov and Natalia Gavrilov, Harwood Academic Publishers, 1991.

Biomarkers by William Evans and Irwin Rosenberg, Simon & Schuster, 1991.

Building a Champion by Bill Walsh, St. Martin's Press, 1990.

The Celebration of Life by Norman Cousins, Harper & Row, 1974.

Centenarians: The New Generation by Belle Boone Beard, Greenwood Press, 1991.

Complete Guide to Aging and Health edited by Mark Williams, M.D., Harmony Books, 1995.

Complexity: Life at the Edge of Chaos by Roger Lewin, Macmillan, 1992.

Creating Minds by Howard Gardner, Basic Books, 1993.

Darwin's Dangerous Idea by Daniel Dennett, Simon & Schuster, 1995.

Don't Forget: Easy Exercises for a Better Memory at Any Age by Danielle Lapp, Simon & Schuster, 1987.

Excellence by John Gardner, W. W. Norton, 1978.

Flow by Mihaly Csikszentmihaly, HarperCollins, 1990.

The Fountain of Age by Betty Friedan, Simon & Schuster, 1993.

A Fresh Map of Life by Peter Laslett, Harvard University Press, 1991.

Growing Old Is Not for Sissies by Etta Clark, Pomegranate Art Books, 1986.

Healthwise Handbook by Donald Kemper, Kathleen McIntosh, and Toni Roberts, Healthwise, 1991.

Helplessness: On Depression, Development and Death by Martin Seligman, Freeman & Sons, 1974.

How and Why We Age by Leonard Hayflick, Ballantine, 1994.

Human Options by Norman Cousins, W. W. Norton, 1981.

Living to Be 100 by Osborne Segerberg, Scribner's, 1982.

Longevity, Senescence, and the Genome by Caleb E. Finch, University of Chicago Press, 1990.

Man's Search for Meaning by Viktor Frankl, Simon & Schuster, 1984.

Mathematics and Optimal Form by Stefan Hildebrandt and Anthony Tromba, Scientific American Library, 1988.

Maximum Life Span by Roy Walford, W. W. Norton, 1983.

Measuring Functioning and Well-Being by Anita Stewart and John Ware, Duke University Press, 1992.

Mercer Guide to Social Security and Medicare by Dale Detlef, Robert Meyers, and Robert Treavor, William Mercer, Inc., 1994.

Mindfulness by Ellen Langer, Addison Wesley, 1989.

The Mind's Sky by Timothy Ferris, Bantam, 1992.

The New Aerobics by Kenneth Cooper, M. Evans & Company, 1970.

Not In Our Genes: Biology, Ideology, and Human Nature by Richard Lewontin, Stephen Rose, and Leon Kamin, Pantheon, 1984.

Older and Wiser by Gretchen Dianda and Betty Hoffmeyer, Ballantine, 1995.

On Growth and Form by D'Arcy Thompson, Cambridge University Press, 1963.

Order Out of Chaos by Ilya Prigogine and Isabelle Stengers, Bantam, 1984.

The Phenomenon of Man by Teilhard de Chardin, Harper Brothers, 1959.

Practical Handbook of Human Biologic Age Determination edited by Arthur K. Bailin, CRC Press, 1994.

Recipes for Your Heart's Delight, Stanford Center for Disease Prevention, 1989.

Retirement Places Rated by David Savageau, Simon & Schuster, 1995.

Retirement Rights: The Benefits of Growing Older by Nancy Levititin, Avon, 1994.

Running Through Life by Paul Spangler, Fifty Plus Fitness Association, 1995.

Self-Renewal by John Gardner, W. W. Norton, 1981.

Setting Limits: Medical Goals in an Aging Society by Daniel Callahan, Simon & Schuster, 1987.

Shadows of Forgotten Ancestors by Carl Sagan and Anne Druyan, Ballantine, 1992.

Sleep Watchers by William Dement, Portable Stanford Press, 1992.

The Social Foundations of Thought in Action by Albert Bandura, Prentice-Hall, 1986.

Stanford Guide to Eating Well: Food for Health, Stanford Center for Research and Disease Prevention, 1990.

Successful Aging edited by Paul Baltes and Margaret Baltes, Cambridge University Press, 1990.

Take Care of Yourself by Donald Vickery and James Fries, Addison Wesley, 1990.

Time's Arrow, Time's Cycle by Stephen J. Gould, Harvard University Press, 1987.

Total Living by Ron Clarke, Pavillion Books Ltd., 1995.

Twelve Steps to a Worry-Free Retirement by David Kehrer, Kiplinger, 1995.

Vital Involvement in Old Age by Erik Erikson, Joan Erikson, and Helen Kivnick, W. W. Norton, 1986.

Vitality in Aging by James Fries and Lawrence Crapo, Freeman & Sons, 1981.

Who Shall Live? by Victor Fuchs, Basic Books, 1974.

The Wisdom of the Ego by George Vaillant, Harvard University Press, 1991.

Resources

AARP, 601 E Street NW, Washington, DC 20049; 202-434-2277

AARP Pharmacy Service, 500 Montgomery Street, Alexandria, VA 22314; 800-456-4036

Administration on Aging, 330 Independence Avenue SW, Washington, DC 20201; 202-619-0724

Aerobics and Fitness Foundation, 15250 Ventura Boulevard, Suite 310, Sherman Oaks, CA 91403; 800-BE-FIT-86

Aging Network Services, 4400 East West Hwy, Bethesda, MD 20814; 301-657-7829

Alcohol, Drug Abuse and Mental Health Administration, 5600 Fisher's Lane, Parklawn Bldg. 12-105, Rockville, MD 20857; 301-443-4797

Alzheimer's Association, 919 N. Michigan Avenue, Chicago, IL 60611; 800-272-3900

Alzheimer's Disease Education Referral Center, Box 8250, Silver Springs, MD 20907; 800-438-4380

American Association of Homes for the Aging, 901 E Street NW, Washington, DC 20004; 202-783-2242

American Cancer Society, 1599 Clifton Road NE, Atlanta, GA 30329; 800-227-2345

American College of Surgeons, 55 E. Erie Street, Chicago, IL 60611; 312-664-4070

American Diabetes Association, 1660 Duke Street, Alexandria, VA 22314; 800-DIA-BETS

American Dietetic Association, 216 W. Jackson Boulevard, Suite 800, Chicago, IL 60606; 800-366-1655

American Federation of Home Health Agencies, 1320 Fenwick Lane, Suite 100, Silver Springs, MD 20910; 301-588-1454

American Foundation for the Blind, 15 W. 16th Street, New York, NY 10011; 800-232-5463

American Geriatrics Society, 770 Lexington Avenue, #300, New York, NY 10021; 212-308-1414

American Heart Association, 7272 Greenville Avenue, Dallas, TX 75231; 800-AHA-USA1

American Hospital Association, 840 N. Lakeshore Drive, Chicago, IL 60611; 800-242-2626

American Lung Association, 1740 Broadway, New York, NY 10019; 212-315-8700

American Medical Association, 515 State Street, Chicago, IL 60610; 800-202-3211

American Nursing Association, 2420 Pershing Road, Kansas City, MO 64108; 800-444-5720

American Parkinson's Disease Association, 60 Bay Street, #401, Staten Island, NY 10301; 800-223-2732

American Red Cross, 18 D Street NW, Washington, DC 20006; 202-737-8300

American Society on Aging, 853 Market Street, San Francisco, CA 94103; 415-882-2912

Arthritis Foundation, 1314 Spring Street, Atlanta, GA 30309; 800-283-7800

Be Fit Networks Personal Trainers; 800-856-2348

Better Hearing Institute, Box 1840, Washington, DC 20013; 800-EAR-WELL

Centers for Disease Control, Office of Public Affairs, 1600 Clifton Road NE, Atlanta, GA 30383; 404-639-3311

Citizens Education and Research Center, 925 15th Street NW, Washington, DC 20005; 202-347-8800

Earthwatch; 800-776-0188

Elder Treks, 597 Markham Street, Toronto, Ontario, Canada M6G 2L7; 800-741-7956

Eldercare Locator; 800-677-1116

Elderhostel, 75 Federal Street, Boston, MA 02110; 617-426-7788

FDA Office of Consumer Affairs, 5600 Fisher's Lane E88, Rockville, MD 20837; 301-443-3170

Fifty Plus Fitness Association, Box D, Stanford, CA 94309; 415-323-6160

Food and Nutrition Information Center, 10301 Baltimore Blvd., #304, Department of Agriculture NALB, Beltsville, MD 20705-2351

Food Safety Hotline, U.S. Department of Agriculture; 800-535-4555

Gerontologic Society of America, 1275 K Street NW, Suite 350, Washington, DC 20005; 202-842-1275

Gray Panthers, 3635 Chestnut Street, Philadelphia, PA 19104

Greetings Office, the White House, Washington, DC 20500; 202-456-1111

Legal Services for the Elderly, 130 W. 42nd Street, 17th Floor, New York, NY 10036; 212-391-0120

National Aging Resource Center on Elder Abuse, 810 First Street NE, Suite 500, Washington, DC 20002; 202-682-2476

National Alliance for Senior Citizens, 1700 18th Street NW, Washington, DC 20009; 202-986-0117

National Arthritis and Musculoskeletal Diseases Information Clearinghouse, Box AMS, 9000 Rockville Pike, Bethesda, MD 20910; 301-495-4484

National Association for Home Care, 519 C Street NE, Washington, DC 20002; 202-547-7424

National Association of Area Agencies on Aging, 1112 16th Street NW, Washington, DC 20036; 202-296-8130

National Association of Meal Programs, 100 N. Alfred Street, Alexandria, VA 22314; 703-548-5558

National Cancer Institute, Cancer Information Service, 9000 Rockville Pike, Bethesda, MD 20852; 800-422-6237

National Caucus and Center on Black Aged, 1424 K Street NW, Washington, DC 20005; 202-637-8400

National Citizens Coalition for Nursing Home Reform, 1426 16th Street NW, Washington, DC 20036; 202-332-2275

National Council on Aging, 409 Third Street SW, Washington, DC 20024; 202-479-1200

National Council on Alcoholism, 1210 21st Street, New York, NY 10010; 212-206-6730

National Council on Senior Citizens, 1331 F Street NW, Washington, DC 20004; 202-347-8800

National Eye Institute, Information Office, Building 31, Room 6A32, 31 Center Drive, MSC 2510, Bethesda, MD 20892-2510; 301-496-5248

National Heart, Lung and Blood Institute, Box 3010, Bethesda, MD 20824; 301-251-1222

National Hospice Organization, 1901 North Moore Street, Suite 901, Arlington, VA 22209; 703-343-5900

National Institute on Aging, Box 8057, Gaithersburg, MD 20857; 800-222-2225

National Institute on Deafness and Other Communication Disorders, Information Office, Building 31, Room 3C35, 9000 Rockville Pike, Bethesda, MD 20852; 301-496-7243

National Institute on Neurological Disorders and Stroke, 31 Center Drive, NSC 2540, Bethesda, MD 20892; 800-352-9424

National Osteoporosis Foundation, 1150 17th Street NW, Suite 500, Washington, DC 20036

National Rehabilitation Information Center, 8455 Colesville Road, Suite 935, Silver Springs, MD 20910; 508-227-0216

National Senior Citizens Law Center, 1815 H Street NW, Suite 700, Washington, DC 20006; 202-887-5280

National Society to Prevent Blindness, 500 E. Remington Road, Schaumberg, IL 60173; 800-331-2020

National Stroke Association, 300 East Hampden Avenue, Englewood, CO 80110; 303-762-9922

Nursing Home Information Service, National Council of Senior Citizens Education and Research Center, 925 15th Street NW, Washington, DC 20005; 202-347-8800

Office of Disease Prevention and Health Promotion, National Health Information Center, Box 1132, Washington, DC 20013; 800-336-4797

Older Adult Service and Information System (OASIS), 7710 Carondelet, Suite 125, St. Louis, MO 63105; 314-862-2933

Older Americans Volunteer Programs Office, 1100 Vermont Avenue NW, 6th Floor, Washington, DC 20525; 202-606-1855

President's Council on Physical Fitness and Sport, 701 Pennsylvania Avenue NW, Suite 250, Washington, DC 20004; 202-272-3430

Senior Net, 399 Arguello, San Francisco, CA 94188; 415-750-5030

Senior Ventures Network, Sikiyou Center, South Oregon State College, Ashland, OR 97520; 800-257-0577

Service Corps of Retired Executives, Small Business Administration, 409 Third Street, SW, Washington, DC 20024; 202-205-6762

United Parkinson's Foundation, 833 W. Washington Blvd., Chicago, IL 60607; 312-733-1893

United Seniors Health Cooperative, 1331 8th Street NW, Washington, DC 20005; 202-393-6222

Vestibular Disorders Association, P.O. Box 4467, Portland, OR 97208; 503-229-7705

Visiting Nurse Associations of America, 3801 E. Florida Avenue, Suite 206, Denver, CO 80200; 800-426-2547

Willard Scott, *Today,* 30 Rockefeller Plaza, Suite 352, New York, NY 10112; 212-664-5488